Needs Assessment in Public Health

A Practical Guide
for Students and Professionals

Needs Assessment in Public Health

A Practical Guide
for Students and Professionals

Donna J. Petersen

and

Greg R. Alexander

School of Public Health
University of Alabama at Birmingham
Birmingham, Alabama

Springer Science+Business Media, LLC

Library of Congress Cataloging-in-Publication Data

Petersen, Donna J.
    Needs assessment in public health: a practical guide for students and professionals
Donna J. Petersen and Greg R. Alexander.
        p.   cm.
    Includes bibliographical references and index.
    ISBN 978-1-4757-7447-4   ISBN 978-0-306-47610-5 (eBook)
    DOI 10.1007/978-0-306-47610-5
    1. Public health.   2. Needs assessment.   3. Community health services.   I. Alexander,
Greg R.   II. Title.

RA425 .P38 2001
362.1—dc21

                                                                    00-052733

ISBN 978-1-4757-7447-4

©2001 Springer Science+Business Media New York
Originally published by Kluwer Academic / Plenum Publishers, New York in 2001
Softcover reprint of the hardcover 1st edition 2001

http://www.wkap.nl/

10 9 8 7 6 5 4 3 2

A C.I.P. record for this book is available from the Library of Congress

Preface

This book has been designed to serve both as a textbook for public health students and as a handbook for public health practitioners interested in improving their understanding and skills in the area of needs assessment. The *assessment* function of public health is essential in the development of appropriate policy and programmatic solutions to persistent and emergent public health concerns, yet few public health professionals are adequately trained in these activities. It is hoped this resource will not only provide a sufficient foundation for those who will lead or participate in needs assessments and related efforts in the future, but also engender a level of enthusiasm for the collection, analysis, and interpretation of data in the pursuit of public health goals.

Given this dual purpose as textbook and handbook, the chapters follow the typical sequence of an actual needs assessment process, from conceptualization of the task through the application of needs-based data to effective public health solutions. The book begins with three case examples which will be referred to throughout the text; these are completely fictional and meant to illustrate the strengths and weaknesses of needs assessment activities observed or experienced by the authors over the past decade. The book also describes the cyclic nature of needs assessment, the need to build sustainable teams of knowledgeable professionals engaged in relevant tasks at various points in time, and the ways in which needs assessments are most effectively communicated, utilized, and promoted toward sound public health policy and programs. We draw examples from myriad public health efforts, recognizing that not all public sector health agencies bear direct responsibility for all activities that could be considered part of public health. We hope you find this text enlightening and enjoyable. Happy learning!

Acknowledgments

In any worthwhile endeavor, the support of dedicated people is critical to accomplishing the task at hand. The development of this textbook is no exception. The ideas contained in this book have evolved through several different efforts on the part of the authors. In the early 1990s, we were invited to develop and present a series of workshops on needs assessment for state maternal and child health programs around the country. At the same time, we began to develop a curriculum around needs assessment for public health graduate students. These parallel efforts coalesced beautifully thanks to the particular efforts of Ms. Jodi Eieseland and Ms. Margaret Ruble Celebrezze, who at the time were graduate students in public health at the University of Minnesota. As we began to pull this textbook together, we sought and received help from one of our UAB School of Public Health alumnae, Ms. Michelle Bajjalieh, and an undergraduate student from Princeton, Ms. Rebecca Pass, both of whom were instrumental in identifying pertinent reference material and in giving the unfolding text the "student eye." Finally, in the last stages of assembling the finished product we enlisted the competent assistance of one of our current UAB graduate students, Ms. Martha Slay. To each of these women we are indebted, not only for their capable assistance, but also for their ability to motivate us to make this guide to needs assessment in public health the best it could possibly be.

Contents

1

The Context for Needs Assessment
Past, Present, and Future

Introduction

Public health is an interesting creature. While public health embodies a set of activities critical to the healthy development and quality of life of people around the world, the term "public health" is poorly understood. Few may fully appreciate the effort required to undertake its responsibilities.

A 1995 Harris Poll confirmed what many in public health already believed: The general public does not know what public health is (Taylor, 1997). Notwithstanding, they do know and care deeply about some of the things it does. The reasons for the incongruous public view of public health are difficult to discern and remain open to debate. The unique history of the development of private medicine in the United States may partially underlie the current public opinion on the role and importance of public health, along with our nation's ongoing mixed feelings about the role of government in health care matters.

In 1988, the Institute of Medicine defined public health as creating those conditions in which people can be healthy in order to advance society's collective interest in promoting and preserving good health (IOM, 1988). This societal interest is best served if:

- The air, food, and water supply remain safe.
- The medical care system functions efficiently and effectively.
- Communities work together to support the optimal growth and development of all children and families and promote quality of life across the life span.
- Workplaces, schools, and recreation sites are safe.

- People engage in healthy lifestyle choices that prolong a high-quality life.
- Appropriate and necessary services and supports are designed and maintained to meet community and individual needs for physical, mental, and spiritual health.

The Institute of Medicine's phrase "creating those conditions in which people can be healthy" is another way of saying "doing whatever it takes to prevent unnecessary disease, disability, or premature death." Because of public health's emphasis on prevention, it is virtually invisible when it is most successful in performing its duties and achieving its goals. When water and food are safe to consume, the air is clean, sewage is treated, and people are relatively free of disease, it is easy for the public to forget that these blessings just don't happen. Instead, they are the products of the ongoing endeavors of the many disciplines of public health.

In recent years, public health has engaged in broader efforts to promote health beyond the prevention of disease. This is consistent with the World Health Organization definition of health as a complete state of physical, mental, and social well-being and not merely the absence of disease or infirmity. Whether focused on the prevention of disease or the promotion of health at the individual, institutional, or community level, the mission of public health requires many people from multiple disciplines working together toward a set of agreed upon health goals. This in turn depends on a well-articulated set of objectives toward which resources can be directed and success monitored. The determination of public health objectives, which the public and policymakers view as obtainable, realistic, and important, ultimately depends on the availability of empirical data to support decision-making. For needs assessment, data and opinions are used in a process that establishes a public consensus regarding the current public health concerns and priorities, as well as the most cost-effective strategies to address them.

Since the early days of public health, data and statistical indicators have been used to identify and define problems. While it may be more common to view public health's use of data as part of its disease investigation and epidemiological research functions, data-based indicators contribute to every stage of the public health planning cycle from needs analysis and problem identification to monitoring, evaluating, and measuring performance (Fig. 1.1).

For some public health programs, like those authorized under Title V of the Social Security Act (U.S. Congress, 1935) and those supported by the Pre-

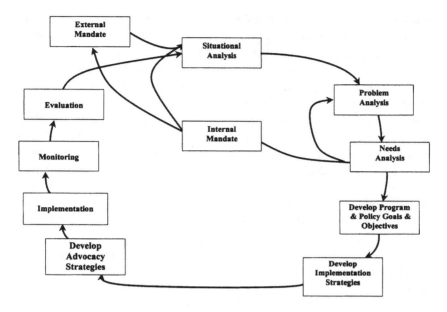

Figure 1.1. The planning, implementation, and evaluation model.

ventive Health and Health Services Block Grant (U.S. Congress, 1981), state health agencies are required to engage in periodic needs assessments toward the development of plans that achieve national and state health objectives. Historically, needs assessment has served federal, state, and local public health agencies as the foundation for the development of programmatic and policy directives and for the allocation of resources to achieve strategic objectives. In recognition of the importance of these activities, the Institute of Medicine, in the same report that articulated the mission of public health, identifies *assessment* as one of the three core functions of public health, the other two being policy development and assurance, both of which rest on the success or failure of assessment efforts (IOM, 1988)

The public health assessment function is described as the responsibility of every public health agency to "regularly and systematically collect, assemble, analyze and make available information on the health of the community, including statistics on health status, community health needs and epidemiologic and other studies of health problems" (IOM, 1988, p. 7). While this may suggest a more traditional surveillance role, reporting on births and deaths, communicable diseases, environmental hazards, and incidence of cancer, public health actually adopts a broader perspective and considers not only the immediate causes of disease or premature death but also the social, economic, cultural, and health care system factors that predispose to ill health or that promote a longer quality of life. This view suggests four key components as cornerstones for the development of a broad public health surveillance system that can inform needs assessment efforts. These components entail the concepts of (1) health status, (2) health service utilization, (3) health systems, and (4) population/contextual characteristics. Their hypothesized relationships to one another can be characterized in a conceptual, causal model (Fig. 1.2).

The health status of a population is directly impacted by current patterns of health care utilization, the existing health system, and population and contextual factors. As illustrated in the model, the prevailing health status will reciprocally influence observed patterns of health service utilization, potentially impact the attributes of the health system through societal responses toward the development of systems to meet recognized and changing health status needs, and will influence, both in the short and long term, population characteristics. Moreover, there is an interrelationship among the three precursors of health status. Population characteristics contribute to the development and nature of the health system. The availability and attributes of a health system directly influence the population characteristics of the surrounding community. Both of these components further influence health care utilization. Although health care utilization may be viewed as an attribute of the health care system, a separate treatment of this concept is proposed on the grounds that utilization, while being influenced by the health system, is an expressed behavior of the population and, as such, may be equally influenced by distinct population characteristics. There is also a reciprocal relationship between utilization and the characteristics of a health system and the population. Variations in utilization (demand) may effect changes in the health system (supply) and eventually impact the nature of the population.

It is evident that needs assessment efforts can no longer be viewed as restricted to the compilation and consideration of solely health status measures. Given that the role of needs assessment is to identify and also address needs, needs assessment efforts therefore must give recognition to the influence of health care system attributes, as well as population characteristics, on health status and include measures of the health care system and the population into its process. As ameliorating pressing health status needs often requires addressing health care utilization and system issues, the inclusion of

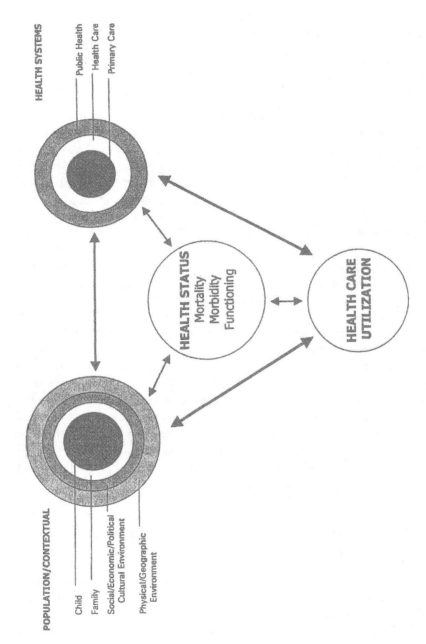

Figure 1.2. Public health surveillance system model.

these elements is critical to the ultimate goal of needs assessment: improving, promoting, and protecting the health status of the public.

Assessing the Needs of All

As we enter the new millennium, we are devoting more and more attention to system reforms across multiple sectors including health care, welfare, education, tele-communications, environmental protection, and government, among others. Particularly in this era of continuing system reform, it is appropriate and critical for the public health sector to assess the impact of such reforms on the health of the public. Reforms in the nation's health care financing and delivery systems have brought to clarity questions regarding the full scope of public health's assessment function. Despite the failure of the Clinton Health Plan in the early years of the Clinton presidency, interest in cost containment, improved access, and increased quality of health care have led to health system reforms. These have been the result of state legislative or regulatory intervention, incremental steps by Congress (e.g., the Health Portability and Coverage Act of 1996), and market-driven changes, including mergers, the creation of integrated networks, and the development of various payment and benefits packages. The rapid escalation and evolution in health care reform over the past decade has had a substantial impact on public health activities at state and local levels in several ways. Many constituencies who once relied mainly on pubic health for direct health care services now find themselves receiving health care in managed care arrangements, including those whose care is covered in the private sector by their employers and those who have public coverage through Medicare (federal health insurance coverage for citizens over 65) and Medicaid (federal–state health insurance coverage for persons of low income or with chronic medical conditions).

This large-scale movement of persons who had previously received care through publicly funded clinics into new health care arrangements as well as the elimination of public health's access to revenues from Medicaid fee-for-service dollars has challenged public health to reconsider its role in providing medical services. Moreover, it has brought attention to the question of just who is public health's service population and who should be the users of the results of public health's needs assessment efforts. In regard to needs assessment, this book takes the position that public health is responsible for assessing the health needs of the entire population, regardless of their source or payer of health care services. Further, this responsibility includes the publication and dissemination of the results of the assessment for the use of all interested parties.

Managed care health plans differ fundamentally from traditional fee-for-service insurance coverage in several ways that are relevant to needs assessment efforts. One difference of particular interest to public health is managed care's shift in emphasis away from expensive medical treatments for existing diseases toward the prevention of disease occurrence. This emphasis on prevention provides tremendous opportunities for partnership between public health and health plans, whether publicly or privately organized, who also view disease prevention as a primary goal. The prevention focus has also led some health plans to venture outside of traditional patient-directed clinical responsibilities and into the area of community-based prevention interventions, again providing opportunities for collaboration with public health. Desires by health plans and provider networks to improve community health or at least the health of the communities of their service populations have simultaneously generated their interest in undertaking community needs assessments.

The opportunities for coordination and partnership between health plans and public health on assessments of community health needs are increasingly apparent and the benefits of such are fairly obvious. However, these potential joint private sector/public health efforts may be frustrated by a number of potential conflicts. The organizational missions of public health and private health plans may vary widely, differing from meeting the health care needs of enrollees while increasing dividends to stockholders, to promoting and protecting the health of the entire public. The definitions of the target population may also differ from enrollees residing in a specific service catchment area to the entire population of a community. Moreover, health plan coverage areas vary widely and often overlap, while government public health agencies typically follow geopolitical boundaries or jurisdictions, such as cities or counties. These innate dissimilarities between public health and health care plans can result in separate foci of their assessment efforts and disparate expectations surrounding the process. While entities interested in "health," however perceived, could ideally work together in the design and conduct of needs assessments, this is not the normal case. At a minimum, needs assessment activities should be communicated across agencies, reports should be shared, and the potential for data sharing should be explored.

For population-based needs assessment efforts, a positive aspect of the growth of managed care products, in which the financing and the delivery of health care are handled by a single entity (the "health plan"), has been the development of large comprehensive databases on all health plan enrollees that include information on enrollment status, service utilization, and reimbursement claims. These databases have the potential to provide a wealth of information previously unavailable on large populations across communities, though concerns for patient confidentiality and protection of privacy have introduced an appropriate level of caution into efforts to fully exploit these databases even for what some believe are laudable purposes.

Because of public health's assessment function, which includes not only identifying new health concerns but also monitoring overall health status, the importance of attending to the effects, intended or otherwise, of health care system reforms on the health of the public cannot be overstated. As attributes of the health care system are critical determinants of the population's health status, the monitoring of the functioning, health, and potential for system failure of the health care system cannot be totally divorced from needs assessment. The successes of health reforms in slowing the growth in health care expenditures, in containing cost, and in improving access to care, in terms of both health insurance coverage and utilization of health services, are fundamental questions for needs assessments, as are the assessment of changes in health care quality, content, appropriateness, and population coverage, e.g., determining coverage under Medicare, Medicaid, or other publicly financed health plans. Finally, needs assessment efforts must consider the possible differential impact of health care reform on specific population subgroups and explore whether some population groups experienced enhanced health at the expense of others. This entails assessing subgroup population disparities in health status, health care use and access, and determining whether the particular needs of vulnerable populations are being adequately addressed.

Though the interests of vulnerable populations have long been at the forefront of public health efforts, public health supports everyone's interests in maintaining good health and a positive quality of life. This broader focus is often lost in political and public debate around the roles and responsibilities of public health, for everyone, regardless of social or economic circumstances, is vulnerable to disease, injury, disability, or premature death whether due to adverse conditions in the home, community, or work environment, imprudent lifestyle and behavior choices, inherited biologic or genetic factors, or deficiencies in available health care services. As such, public health assumes responsibility for assessing, monitoring, and correcting or enhancing those conditions, behaviors, or systems that affect the health of the population or subpopulations, positively or negatively.

Because many sectors of the population do not enjoy the same "conditions in which people can be healthy," it is incumbent on public health to pay special attention to vulnerable populations: the elderly; pregnant women and children including adolescents and those with special health care needs; persons with disabilities; families living below the federal poverty level; immigrants; and persons living in isolation whether that be in sparsely populated rural areas or decaying urban neighborhoods. These vulnerable populations are most susceptible to the unanticipated consequences of policies, programs, and institutions that are not always designed to accommodate the unique needs of these groups. As such, the assessment function of public health must not only consider the needs of the many, it must ensure that the needs of vulnerable groups are also regularly assessed and given attention.

Toward Accountability and Performance

Public demands for accountability and clear documentation of outcomes achieved for dollars spent have led to congressional efforts to shift reporting emphasis away from process measures of service delivery, e.g., clinic visits or encounters, toward outcome measures of actual improvement, e.g., health status attainment. The movement toward performance measurement for public programs is codified in the Government Performance and Results Act of 1993, which requires every federal program to develop a system to report on annual performance and achievement of performance goals (U.S. Congress, 1993) Suddenly, the customary data collected and the indicators derived take on new importance as they are used not only to document population need but also to assess whether or not specific or collective efforts have succeeded or failed. A persistent high rate of infant mortality that once led to special program funding may now be used to reallocate funding, which may penalize some programs by potentially reducing their traditional funding levels.

The choice of indicators, whether of need or of performance, is a political process. This should not be surprising when the functions of needs assessment and accountability are inherently political and require the participation of a broad constituency base. The sources of data for needs or for performance are limited. Therefore, states are being challenged to consider new ways of garnering needed information, e.g., linking existing data sets, developing new partnerships with other public or private agencies to share data of mutual interest, or even developing new primary data collection strategies. However public health agencies choose to respond, the level of change in systems that affect the lives of vulnerable populations, the growth in the demands for limited and rational allocation of resources, and the need for clear lines of responsibility, compel public health to greatly enhance its capacity to gather, utilize, interpret, and report data. Many believe that such improvement is long overdue.

We view needs assessment as an essential component of an ongoing planning cycle that has no beginning and no end. However, many planning efforts are initiated by some event, be it the creation of a new mandate, the availability of funds, the reorganization of an agency, the recruitment of new leadership, or the routine development of proposals linked to legislative or budgetary cycles. Regardless of what triggers planning efforts, they are enormously enhanced by successful needs assessments. In this way, needs assessment can be viewed as one of the earliest steps in the planning cycle and so it behooves public health professionals to be familiar with needs assessment methodologies and models; to maintain an active and ongoing needs assessment agenda; and to have available resources, including human, technical, and financial, with which to engage in broad-based or targeted needs assessments. The following chapters in this textbook are designed to provide guidance in the conduct of periodic or ongoing needs assessments, beginning with steps in the needs assessment process and sources of data and continuing through communicating needs assessment data, determining priorities, and setting goals and objectives and ending with the link to planning, monitoring, and evaluation efforts so critical to successful public health interventions.

Hypothetical Case Examples

To illustrate the varying approaches to needs assessment taken by state public health agencies in the United States and to provide a context for the discussion questions provided at the end of each chapter in this book, we have contrived three needs assessment scenarios for three fictitious states. The States of Old Virginia, New Carolina, and Central Dakota are all planning or undertaking comprehensive needs assessments, using various methods and processes, any of which can be successfully employed in differing situations. We will challenge you to apply what you've learned in each chapter in responding to questions we will pose based on these three case examples. We suggest you review them now and familiarize yourself with each one, and then refer back to them as needed to formulate your answer to each discussion question.

Case Example #1
State of Old Virginia

As the first stage of planning and developing five-year goals and objectives for the state of Old Virginia, staff in the office of health information assembled available data from every unit in the health department. These data were drawn from such sources as vital statistics (birth and death data), acute disease surveillance and the immunization registry, hospital discharge and injury E-codes, birth defects and genetics registries, federally funded periodic surveys (Behavioral Risk Factor Surveillance System, Youth Risk Behavior Survey, and Pregnancy Risk Assessment Monitoring System), and program participation databases (e.g., breast and cervical cancer screening, WIC, prenatal and well-child clinics, children with special health needs treatment services). Commonly used indicators and trend data were drawn from these data sources and compiled into a "health profile" document, one for the state as a whole and separate profiles for each county and health district in the state.

These health profiles were sent to county and district health departments to provide a basis for local needs assessments. Training sessions were held regionally across the state for local and district health department staff to assist in data interpretation and to suggest strategies for gathering additional information at the local level. Within the state health department, key staff from each unit were asked to provide their own program-specific goals and objectives using the data provided in the health profile as well as their insights into particular areas of need and future program developments.

At the local level, health leaders were given flexibility to conduct their needs assessments as they wished, given their understanding of their local community, health system, and citizen culture. Some arranged town meetings, others assembled steering committees of key leaders and health professionals, others used focus groups of providers, community leaders and clients, while still others used data from previous assessment efforts and formed in-house teams to develop long-range plans. From these various assessment efforts, local plans were developed and submitted to the state for compilation into an overall state plan. State goals were selected based on the frequency with which areas of need emerged from the local assessments and were included in local plans, and on the areas of greatest importance determined by state health department officials.

The state of Old Virginia Five Year Public Health Plan was presented to the legislature as part of the Department's budget request, was distributed to local health officials at the state's annual public health conference, and was placed on the Internet to ensure full public access to the document. As always, public comment was invited.

Case Example #2
State of New Carolina

The newly appointed Health Commissioner of the State of New Carolina embarked on her agency's five-year planning process by creating a new unit responsible for community assessment and planning. This unit recruited and placed staff in regional offices throughout the state in addition to assembling skilled data analysts, community organizers, and communications experts at the state level. Each local unit was asked to assign one or more representatives to the overall effort; a retreat was held and the plan for a community-based statewide needs assessment was determined.

Based on knowledge of local communities, key informants were identified to serve on local assessment committees. Based on the input of these groups within each community, a series of events were organized to maximize citizen participation in the discussion of health-related community needs and the identification of possible solutions. Existing community groups were approached; focus groups were arranged; schools, employers, churches, and recreational sites were visited; and with the help of local media, well-publicized town meetings were held in communities across the state. Participants and responders in each of these sessions were asked how they felt about the quality of their individual lives and of their community as a whole; they were asked to share their perceptions of the overall health of the members of their community and to identify key factors affecting health, positively or negatively; they were asked about the physical environment, the political environment, the health care system as well as what they believed to be the effectiveness of public health efforts to protect them from disease, disability, or premature death. They were asked for ideas on how best to tackle identified health concerns.

Information gleaned from these local efforts was tabulated for interpretation and recommendations from the local assessment team; these were submitted to the regional teams for compilation at the multicounty level; persistent themes were highlighted and individual needs within particular areas were also noted. All of this information was then assembled for state-level analysis; staff of the various units were asked to identify sources of data to support the themes and particular needs identified by the communities. Staff of the state Center for Health Statistics developed a supporting data document to further explicate the problems noted by community members.

The Commissioner is now asking all of her unit heads and each local health officer to review their existing programs and objectives in light of this community-based needs assessment. Given the resources available (human, financial, and technical), she has asked for revised plans that she will take back to the community assessment teams for review and comment. Additional public input will be solicited before the plan is finalized.

Case Example #3
State of Central Dakota

The state of Central Dakota was the first to fully embrace health reform, to pursue universal health care coverage for all its citizens, and to seek ways to privatize much of what had been the responsibility of the state public health system. Many of the health plans that now successfully operate within the state enroll significant numbers of previously uninsured people and have worked hard to develop good working relationships with community health agencies to address the particular needs of these populations. In so doing, they have discovered that many of their enrollees could benefit from public health efforts and that some of the problems they treat through medical interventions may have been prevented through public health strategies.

Two of the four largest health plans have approached the state health officer and proposed a joint public/private statewide needs assessment. Based on reviews of their claims data and their collective experience, they believe the focus should be on adolescent pregnancy, domestic violence, and work-site injuries. They have agreed to recruit at their expense experts in each of these three areas in addition to a senior market researcher who will direct the entire effort. They have asked the health officer for additional staff support and for access to data on these issues to inform their efforts. As they collectively have clinic sites in every large area of the state, they propose surveying a random selection of clients on their personal experiences with and perceptions of these problems. They are looking for ideas for community- and employer-based interventions to reduce the incidence of these conditions. They are also particularly interested in what they as health plans can do to combat these costly problems.

The health plans would also like to survey their network providers and would like the health officer to conduct a similar survey of health department officials. They have already spoken with key members of the legislature to build support for possible requests for additional funds or new policy initiatives resulting from this assessment. They have also developed materials on these topics for use in patient education efforts. Finally, they are hoping this partnership can be extended into the actual implementation phase and have begun developing liaison positions to ensure ongoing communication with the health department on these critical issues.

2

The Process of Needs Assessment

Purpose and Intent of Needs Assessment

Needs assessments are undertaken for a number of reasons, most explicit and praiseworthy, some implicit, and others more Machiavellian in nature. For existing programs and agencies, it is appropriate that there be a periodic reappraisal of whether their various services and activities continue to be needed. Such reassessments of needs can serve several purposes. Needs assessment can be used to validate the current target populations in need of services as well as to identify new target populations with unmet needs. For the reestablished target populations, needs assessments can help reaffirm current need priorities and acknowledge new ones. These in turn can be used to refine or redefine appropriate goals, objectives, and activities of programs and agencies and, in some cases, can result in the development of new programs.

Given their many purposes, needs assessments play a vital role in strategic planning, and in program and policy development efforts. Moreover, needs assessments, by incorporating a review of both the need for services and an assessment of the effectiveness of past operations aimed at meeting those needs, can also be used to maintain or transform program and service philosophies and organizational structures. Needs assessment results can offer useful information for a wide range of reorganizational considerations, including organizational placement of programs within an agency, service delivery approaches (e.g., direct service versus contractual arrangements), and the extent to which centralized versus decentralized management strategies should be used.

Underlying the many uses for needs assessment information is the understanding that the results may bring about marked changes. Needs assessment results not only can alter perceptions regarding the need for an activity, program, or agency, but also can reshape a program's purpose, direction, organization, operations, and personnel complement. The potentially far-reaching, unpredictable, and tumultuous consequences of such changes are disquieting and, in response, there is a predictable tendency on the part of program directors to tightly control the process.

As rapid and ongoing reforms in business, health care, and government during the last few decades have shown, change is the natural order of affairs, despite the human tendency to prefer stability and consistency. Change is often a frightening and difficult thing for organizations and individuals to confront. It is not surprising that needs assessments, which can be used in myriad ways to advocate for a breadth of minor to major changes, are often viewed with apprehension and mixed emotions. Indeed, the announcement that a needs assessment will be undertaken may result in an immediate reaction on the part of program people that someone "higher up" believes they are not doing their job or that their jobs should be eliminated or transferred elsewhere. Alternatively, a call for a needs assessment that originates from within a program may be viewed by those outside the program as little more than a preemptive strike or self-serving attempt to justify the continued existence of an ineffective and inefficient operation or to support the program's expansionary or empire-building schemes.

The many self-serving and conflicting motives that can be attributed to nearly any proposal to undertake a needs assessment are fuel for controversy and criticism, the very threat of which can dissuade such proposals from ever being made. Nevertheless, needs assessment is too vital for strategic leadership to avoid, for without it programs lose focus, effectiveness, and accountability. By establishing internal policies for the routine and ongoing conduct of needs assessment, some of the controversy regarding "motives" can be circumvented. Alternately, external directives for needs assessments that are tied to funding and accountability requirements can also reduce speculation about possible ulterior motives for conducting a needs assessment. Furthermore, external mandates that stipulate the execution of ongoing needs assessments can add credibility to the undertaking. For example, funding to states under the Maternal and Child Health Services Block Grant authorized under Title V, is conditional on the conduct of periodic needs assessments (HRSA, 1999). Without this mandate, it is debatable whether periodic assessments of the health status and service needs of children and their families would be carried out in the United States on a regular basis. And, of those needs assessments that might be implemented, questions would be expected to arise regarding their "real intent."

Whether for new or for existing programs, the fundamental intent of an ongoing needs assessment process should be to help answer the following questions for the program's target population:

- Who is the target population?
- What are the target population's needs?
- Which groups within the target population have these needs?
- Geographically, where are those in need?
- What is currently being done to aid those in need, by whom and where?
- What and where are the unmet needs?
- How well did we do in addressing those needs in the past?
- What has changed since we started?

The very nature of these questions reveals some of the key aspects of the needs assessment process and its intent. First, the questions (and the needs assessment process itself) start with a focus on *who is the target population* and *what are the needs of that population*, not on what the program does. Further, it recognizes that within any target population there is diversity in needs among population subgroups that must be explored and considered. Moreover, it recognizes the importance of geographically locating the target population with specific needs and the existing services that might address those needs, as service delivery site location and availability will influence service and program utilization. Next, the assessment of needs involves exploring what is being done by other programs and agencies in order to arrive at an assessment of unmet need. Only after these questions are resolved does the needs assessment turn its attention to the program. And, it does so for the purpose of self-evaluation of program effectiveness. The final question focuses on change and is a reminder of the importance of returning in the near future to the start of the list. As needs, target populations, resources, and the cost-effectiveness of any service or program are ever-changing, the needs assessment process must be ongoing. It is not a singular goal to be accomplished and checked off the list. Instead, it is a perpetual leadership activity that should be fully integrated into management and administrative practice.

Stepping back and reflecting on the broad intent of needs assessment, a case can be made that needs assessment in the public health arena entails ongoing strategic leadership functions that go far beyond a mere analysis and listing of health status need indicators. Health status assessment and monitoring, program planning, development, implementation and evaluation, and policy analysis and advocacy are all part of the total needs assessment process. When viewed and implemented as an ongoing administrative function, the appropriate motive for needs assessment is apparent: It is to provide and disseminate scientifically credible information to the public, programs, stakeholders, and policymakers that can be used to identify existing and emerging needs and to advocate for and ensure that, when possible, effective and accountable programs, services, and policies are available to meet those needs.

Needs as Values and Policy Statements

Implicit in any needs assessment process is the determination of what are the "needs." But, what is a "need" and how should we define it? Within the context of the needs assessment process, needs are value judgments that suggest that problems exist for target populations (McKillip, 1987). It is also tacit to the needs assessment process that these needs are problems that can in some way be resolved. Hence, the needs assessment process entails three broad basic parts:

- The identification of problems or needs within a specific target population
- The identification of effective, efficient, and socially acceptable solutions to those problems
- Getting those solutions enacted into policy!

The identification of effective, efficient, and socially acceptable solutions and the development of strategies for getting those solutions enacted into policy are topics dealt with in detail in other chapters of this book. It is pertinent to note at this point that these practical considerations must be weighed in any determination of need. Needs must have workable solutions that can be enacted in order to be useful to a needs assessment process that aims to effect constructive change in the health status of populations.

Needs, as statements of the pressing health-related problems of specific target populations, can carry considerable political weight. A well-articulated and documented statement of need can be a powerful catalyst for change, if there is consensus about its importance. In this context, the concept of needs as value judgments is an important one to consider. An individual's assessment of his or her own needs can take on a special reality. Entire hierarchies of needs have been proposed. (Maslow, 1954) Our personal needs do not seem like mere value judgments. Being hungry, sick, unemployed, homeless, or unvalued in society are very real to any individual for whom these basic needs are unmet. But at the population level, defining these same basic needs is less easily done. It becomes less clear who and how many should be defined as hungry, homeless, sick, or in need. Questions of duration, intensity, and intent arise. For example, someone will invariably question whether certain people are hungry, unemployed, and homeless because they refuse to work or to seek assistance. Are some really too sick to work or not? How should we precisely define being hungry or homeless?

Even within the public health profession, uniform agreement about need is unlikely. Consider the following cases and ask yourself if any or all of the groups would be considered top- or low-priority need areas for public health program funding during periods of declining fiscal resources:

- Pregnant teenagers, 18 and 19 years of age, married and living with their spouses
- Incarcerated teenage boys, less than 18 years of age, whose crimes include rape, armed violence, and drug use
- Illegal immigrants
- Native Americans
- High-tech industry workers
- Children with attention deficit hyperactivity disorder
- Seniors living independently

All of the above groups represent potential areas of needs. Some groups, like incarcerated youths, may be less socially attractive to the public, but these children still need preventive health care services for physical, mental, and dental health. High-tech industry workers may not initially appear to be a target audience, but they may be ripe for work-site health promotion programs designed to prevent serious and costly chronic illnesses.

As perceived needs are reflections of personal, cultural, and public values, they are always open to speculation, discussion, and disagreement. Even what might seem the most obvious need to some may not register as important for others. While public health has long been involved in advocating for social justice and addressing the health needs of all populations, public health professionals still routinely fail to reach agreement on need priorities and their importance. Therefore, the first step in preparing for the conduct of a needs assessment is recognizing that needs are not absolute, undisputed, unequivocal, and unchanging. Instead, they start as individual value judgments that apply to defined populations in specific geographic locations during specific time periods. For these multiple individual judgments of need to be useful for program planning and policy development, they must be brought together and discussed in an open forum. Some of these perceptions of need will be met with wide unanimity and will prevail, while others will be discarded for lack of agreement. Ultimately, a public consensus is necessary regarding which perceived needs are so important, unmet, or sufficiently reoccurring that action is warranted.

In order to engender broad public support for needs assessment findings, the analysis of need data and the determination of need priorities should always involve input from the public. Although the identification of public health needs and their priority is often thought of as strictly a scientific process for experts in the health care and public health fields, determining need priorities should be viewed as a political process as well. Moreover, careful attention must be given to identifying the stakeholders who should be involved in needs analysis and determination. Stakeholders are those individuals or groups on which the needs assessment process will directly or indirectly impact. These include:

- The target population and service recipients
- Service providers
- Service funders
- Policymakers
- Members of the community in which the target population and the service provision exist

Who should decide the health-related needs of a population? It can be argued that everyone has a stake. Clearly, public health professionals, as experts in the area, have an opportunity to guide such discussions, but we also have the responsibility to encourage and secure a broad range of input and involvement. Failure to involve a broad base of stakeholders into the initial and subsequent stages of the needs assessment process can have serious consequences that may arise unexpectedly at any stage of the process. If needs are solely determined by the public health professional community, other stakeholders may fail to endorse or support proposed program and policy solutions as either unnecessary, ineffective, duplicative, or just simply unwanted. While public health and health care professionals can often use their educational and professional status in society to sway public opinion or even disregard it, such tactics often backfire in efforts to enact major, far-reaching policy change.

While defining needs in terms of values may suggest that there is little scientific or quantifiable basis for establishing need, this view is not accurate. Statistical indicators of health status, health care system attributes, health care utilization, and socioeconomic and demographic risk characteristics are typically used as a starting point for discussions of need. Statistical indicators provide summary statements about needs that can quickly be grasped and used in discussions. Statistical indicators allow for comparisons across regions and localities, over time periods, and among population subgroups and are heuristic in allowing for policy-level debates regarding need priorities to continue without becoming bogged down in highly personal and fanciful perceptions.

There is considerable merit in using a standard set of indicators that allows for systematic temporal and geographic comparisons. The development of standard indicators further aids in the development and maintenance of ongoing, standardized data collection systems to monitor health needs, population risk characteristics, and the utilization and impact of interventions and service programs. These indicators and indicator data systems facilitate accountability by helping standardize discourse, debate, and analysis, and by aiding in the evaluation of program success. At the same time, the absence of summary need indicators or the lack of a data system to support the ongoing monitoring of indicators can be a serious hindrance to the identification of needs. Not unexpectedly, the public and policymakers are more likely to view as needs those areas for which there are more data available. It is harder to wrap your arms around an issue that cannot be sufficiently defined or quantified.

Without data to substantiate the presence of needs, debates regarding needs become purely speculative, subjective, or even partisan. As such, the needs assessment process is greatly aided by efforts to conceptually define specific need areas, to quantify those needs in terms of statistical indicators, and to develop a standard set of statistical need indicators and a standardized data collection system to support their ongoing measurement. Notwithstanding the importance to the needs assessment process of these seemingly statistical and expert-driven activities, needs assessment remains a political process.

The selection of the statistical indicators and the data sources that will be used to determine needs are political activities in and of themselves. Those who can control which indicators will be developed (or funded for development) and used and who decide what data will be collected on national and state databases, in fact, exert considerable influence over the outcome of the process. A quick review of the indicators that are and are not included in the U.S. Year 2010 Health Objectives is instructive on this point. The selection of data items to collect on national data systems or the removal of requirements for reporting data have profound implications for needs assessment efforts. Accordingly, the processes used to revise the national databases that are heavily relied on for the conduct of public health needs assessments (e.g., the U.S. Census, birth and death records, reportable disease registries) should be of great interest to those who undertake needs assessments. Not collecting information on a topic (e.g., the number of AIDS cases, gunshot wounds, domestic violence, workplace environments) can often have the effect of precluding consideration of the topic as a need area.

As useful as statistical indicators are for needs assessment activities, there is some danger in becoming fixed on specific indicators. Failure to identify new and changing need conditions may allow the available data and indicators to drive the needs assessment process. Due to technological advancements, the importance or relevance of specific need indicators may diminish over time, not keeping pace with the underlying problem being measured. For example, advanced maternal age (>35 years) is no longer a good indicator of risk of infant mortality, as many better-educated, professional women have chosen to delay childbearing. Statistical indicators need to be constantly reviewed with regard to their relevance and outdated ones need to be replaced. However, some indicators may have their own constituencies, with programs and activities geared to the indicators. Accordingly, efforts to abandon or supplant specific need indicators may be met with stiff resistance.

Technological advances may also create changes in the customary interpretation of a trend in a need indicator. For instance, preterm birth rates are rising but this may well be driven more by changes in obstetric practice resulting in earlier intervention to prevent a more adverse outcome, than in any actual increase in the prevalence of risk factors for preterm birth in the population (Alexander *et al.*, 1999). Standard indicators may also not be equivalently relevant to multiple and disparate population subgroups and may provide nonequivalent indicators of risk. As needs assessments efforts become institutionalized, there will be a tendency to interpret need indicators in the same way time after time, which may lead to biased interpretations of need trends and the impact of previous interventions.

Finally, standard need indicators can become the major focus of policy initiatives and may distract focus from the underlying fundamental issues of improving health status and outcomes. Areas without easily constructed or recognized indicators (e.g., mental health) tend to be given less attention or ignored. Other, easily reported indicators (e.g., adolescent pregnancy) consume our attention and may become the "usual suspects" for all problems. The reduction of adolescent pregnancy was included in welfare reform legislation because of the assumption that early birth contributed to a dependence on welfare; the notion that perhaps adolescent pregnancy and welfare dependence were both the result of some other factor was apparently never considered. While standard indicators and indicator data systems are essential to needs assessments, excessive reliance on them to the exclusion of reviewing other sources of information on needs can severely limit the identification of important and emerging needs.

Once again, the choice of need indicators, the use of data sources, and the identification and prioritization of needs is a political process. This should not be surprising when the functions of needs assessment and accountability are inherently political and require the participation of a broad constituency base. The sources of data for needs assessment or for performance measurement are limited. Therefore, public health agencies are being challenged to consider new ways of garnering needed information, e.g., linking existing data sets, developing new partnerships with other public or private agencies to share data of mutual interest, or even developing new primary data collection strategies. However public health agencies choose to respond, the level of change in the health care and social systems that affect the lives of vulnerable populations and the growth in the demands for rational allocation of resources, compel public health to greatly enhance its capacity to gather, utilize, interpret, and report data. Such improvement is long overdue and is still forthcoming.

Types of Needs

Several types of needs exist, but all can usually be defined in terms of *discrepancies between a target state and an actual state*, i.e., what should be versus what is (McKillip, 1987; Kettner *et al.*, 1990; Roth, 1990). We further characterize needs as being *comparative*, defined by experts; *expected, wanted, desired, or felt*, defined by the target population; *expressed*, equivalent to demand for services; or *extrapolated*, derived by applying data from one location to another. *Comparative needs*, or those based on comparisons, are the most commonly used and are typically based on a target state that has been defined by experts. The U.S. Year 2010 Health Objectives are examples of target states defined by experts that geopolitical units (states, counties) can then use in comparison to their own indicators.

Several types of targets can be employed for these comparisons. A target can reflect an ideal state of affairs, a typical or normal level, or a minimum or optimal range. The nation with the highest average life expectancy might be used as an ideal. A state might also compare its life expectancy to other states in its region or to the current U.S. rate. The regional and U.S. rate would be used as norms for comparison. Alternatively, a comparison might be made to the U.S. Year 2010 Health Objectives to establish an optimal target for average life expectancy (another estimated target that was set by experts) or to the 1980 U.S. average life expectancy to set a minimal range, defining an unacceptably low level.

The use of comparisons for generating concern, outrage, and support is a well-established political tool. However, its use is limited to those topics for which data exist from two or more areas. Topics and need areas for which data are not systematically and widely collected are excluded from ready comparisons. Yet, these may be of great importance and should be considered in needs assessment activities. Efforts have been made to extrapolate or estimate statistical need indicators. Formulas have been derived to extrapolate the estimated number of individuals in need of service in one state, using a study from another area as a standard. In the areas of family planning and child health, needs formulas are widely used to determine the discrepancy between those estimated to be in need of service and those currently using the service (Henshaw and Forrest, n.d.; Newacheck, 1991; Newcheck and Taylor, 1992) Debate can still stem from disagreements over the extent to which the proposed formula may produce accurate estimates of needs for service in different parts of the country. Nevertheless, they do allow for comparisons across areas where need indicators on specific topics are not ordinary collected.

Expected, wanted, desired, or felt needs have less typically been considered in public health needs assessment but are a more potent force in getting solutions enacted into policy in the political arena. These types of needs are frequently defined by the target population, the public, policymakers, or stakeholders. These are the needs that people vote for with their feet and their wallets. They reflect the level of dissatisfaction with the discrepancy between the perceived situation and the desired or expected level. These expected levels may be similar to the expectations and desires of the experts or may be viewed as unrealistically high or low by experts. The perceived discrepancies or concerns about existing levels may not be supported by scientific data or opinion, but the demand for action may still be supported in such number and with such fervor that it cannot be ignored.

To the extent that failure to address unmet needs or achieve expected levels of performance results in intense feelings of dissatisfaction among individual stakeholders or the public, growing pressure may emerge to commit new or additional resources to address these needs. That pressure may take the face of demand for new programs or initiatives or the withdrawal of funds from a current program that is viewed as ineffective. When individuals become willing to purchase additional or different services to meet their felt needs or when the public starts voting to raise taxes or voting to elect representatives in support of new legislation or policies, these efforts, aimed at impacting perceived needs, reflect *expressed needs*. The concept of expressed needs is derived from the fields of marketing and economics and encompasses demand for services. Needs assessments that rely solely on comparative needs and do not pay attention to the felt and expressed needs of the public may fail to produce recommendations that are viewed as relevant or in touch with the public sentiment.

Stages in the Needs Assessment Process

Needs assessment represents a multifaceted operation that requires careful planning to ensure its success. Because of the complexities involved, the overall process might best be viewed as a sequence of stages, each of which will need to be planned for and managed. The lack of a detailed initial plan for managing the stages of the needs assessment process can quickly result in overlooking or duplicating vital or costly activities or failing to maintain open communication with stakeholders. In turn, the possible repercussions of poor planning include excessive delays and cost overruns, the loss of stakeholder support, and the eventual forfeiture of the credibility of the entire process. As such, needs assessment efforts require advanced planning and organization with sufficient personnel to ensure their ongoing functioning and direction.

A good initial plan for needs assessment efforts is a fundamental prerequisite for its success. A needs assessment effort is similar to any other project or program. Without a plan that establishes clear goals, objectives, and tasks, sets time lines, identifies key responsibilities of individuals, and allocates adequate resources, the process will likely be unfocused and disorganized. Because needs assessment efforts are inherently political activities, the plan for developing, implementing, managing ,and evaluating the needs assessment effort should be open for scrutiny by all involved in the process. The lack of a detailed initial plan for a needs assessment process or an inability to review this plan are warnings that the process is on shaky ground.

Even though needs assessment is a continuing activity, a description of the process is easier if commenced from a starting point. One means of conceptualizing the activities entailed in the needs assessment process is to view it as a series of essential stages within which there are several key steps, as shown in Table 2.1. Each of the essential stages will be discussed below.

The Start-up Planning Stage

The Start-up Planning Stage provides a perspective and direction to the overall needs assessment effort. It is a good leadership activity and a useful review exercise to review first with staff and then again with the stakeholders who comprise the needs assessment advisory committee (see Chapter 4). The key steps and issues to be addressed in this stage are as follows.

1. Establish the organization structure for the needs assessment

Right from the start, it is crucial to be clear about the organization structure for the needs assessment. This entails identifying who will direct the activity's day-to-day operations and be responsible for their accomplishment. Who are the staff dedicated to this activity? How will stakeholders be involved? Will a needs assessment advisory committee be convened including stakeholders? Will the advisory committee have subcommittees to address specific issues? These are among the key organizational issues to be resolved.

2. Identify the potential uses of the needs assessment

Why are we doing a needs assessment and for whom are we doing it? Even needs assessment efforts that are proscribed by legislative or funding mandates or by agency policy may have unclear rationale and may not fully stipulate how and by whom the results will be used. Reviewing these issues through frank discussions with the staff and stakeholders offers a valuable opportunity to set the proper tone right from the start.

Table 2.1. Stages in the Needs Assessment Process

Start-up Planning Stage
  1. Establish the organization structure for the needs assessment
  2. Identify the potential uses of the needs assessment
  3. Identify the stakeholders of the needs assessment
  4. Identify the overall target population
  5. Identify the types of needs to be assessed
Operational Planning Stage
  1. Establish who will help determine the need indicators and data sources to be considered
  2. Establish who will produce the data reports on the indicators
  3. Determine methodology to be used to rank or prioritize needs in terms of importance
  4. Determine a strategy for organizing and managing meetings
  5. Determine a strategy for managing conflicts and reaching consensus
  6. Determine a strategy for building ongoing coalitions
Data Stage
  1. Identify indicators to characterize need
  2. Identify available data sources
  3. Identify other data needed and a strategy for obtaining them
  4. Identify data to create a Resource Inventory
  5. Assemble data
Needs Analysis Stage
  1. Prioritize needs in terms of importance
  2. Determine subpopulations to which specific needs apply
  3. Identify workable solutions to address needs
  4. Reassess needs in light of available solutions
  5. Identify available resources to meet needs
  6. Reach consensus among stakeholders regarding priority unmet needs and best solutions for specific subpopulations
Program and Policy Development Stage
  1. Develop plans to translate need statements and related solutions into policy
  2. Secure internal agency approval of policy action plans
  3. Communicate results of needs analysis and policy action plans to advocacy groups, the general public, and other agencies
  4. Collaborate and cooperate with advocacy groups and related agencies to foster support for program and policy proposals
  5. Develop plans for monitoring and evaluating your proposed programmatic and policy initiatives when implemented
Resource Allocation Stage
  1. Develop criteria for selection of multiple need indicators
  2. Determine basic tenets to guide the development of funding formulas
  3. Reach consensus among stakeholders on indicators and tenets
  4. Assemble data and construct initial funding formulas
  5. Present formulas to stakeholders and adjust as indicated to reach consensus and broad support

3. Identify the stakeholders of the needs assessment

The political component of the needs assessment process gets going early with the identification and selection of the stakeholders and the individuals who will represent their interests during the process. The identification of stakeholders entails exploring what is at stake for them from this process. Your initial contacts can greatly assist you in identifying other stakeholders who should be involved. As such, there are benefits to keeping the door open at the early stages of the needs assessment. As the process proceeds, it may become more difficult to bring in new members without causing delays and disruption in activities, but if it becomes evident that someone is missing, it is essential that they be invited to participate.

4. Identify the overall target population

In many areas of public health, such as, school health or family planning, the target populations are already well established. For other areas, such as environmental health or disease control, the entire public is the target population. Nevertheless, there is a perception held by some of the public that public health mainly serves the poor and impoverished members of society. It is always useful to discuss who is the target population of the program or agency for which the needs assessment is being conducted. Particularly for programs that have traditional service populations, it is important to reconsider if things have changed and if a different definition of the target population is warranted.

5. Identify the types of need to be assessed

As indicated earlier, most needs assessments rely heavily on the use of comparative need indicators that have been derived from "experts" in the public health field. The consideration of more qualitative data, indicating the expected or felt needs of the populations, is less typical, in part due to the financial and time costs involved in obtaining this information. Attention should be directed during this start-up stage to exploring which types of needs will be assessed, given the money, time, and personnel available. If input is desired regarding the expected needs of the population or the stakeholders, this should be established, planned for, and implemented early in order to avoid delays and to estimate a realistic time line for the needs assessment process.

The Operational Planning Stage

The Operational Planning Stage entails establishing a general strategy for the operations of the needs assessment process. The key steps and issues to be addressed in the stage are as follows and assume an open process involving stakeholders.

1. Establish who will help determine the need indicators and data sources to be considered

Based on the organizational structure of the needs assessment, it should be established and made clear who will be responsible for selecting the need indicators and data sources that will be used in the needs assessment process. There are substantial costs involved in obtaining and calculating values for need indicators by geographic areas and time periods. While ideally needs assessments should consider all possible data, this is not practical. Therefore, there must be a means to maintain the scope of the needs assessment process within manageable and affordable levels. To reduce the potential for controversy regarding those decisions, procedures are needed to define who is responsible for this task and to set the process they will use to carry out this function.

2. Establish who will produce the data reports on the indicators

In the start-up stage, attention was given to establishing an organizational structure for the needs assessment. This involved identifying who would staff the effort. Once a clearer picture has been obtained regarding the types of data sources to be used (see Chapter 3), what kinds of needs will be considered, and what need indicators will be involved, attention should be given to who will produce the data reports on the need indicators. This might be done by internal project staff or in cases that involve the collection of new data, by external professionals hired to design surveys, collect data, and prepare summary reports.

3. Determine the methodology to be used to rank or prioritize needs in terms of importance

Once the reports of the need indicators have been produced, a method for prioritizing needs is needed. It may be unwise to wait until the data reports are available to establish this process. Having available a preestablished and agreed-on procedure for ranking or prioritizing needs may alleviate any concerns of those involved in this aspect of the process regarding how the data will be used. While no method is free of bias, consistency and clarity about the method used can be an asset (see Chapter 4).

4. Determine a strategy for organizing and managing meetings

As establishing consensus regarding need priorities and their solutions is a potentially difficult operation, several meetings may be necessary to accomplish these tasks. To keep the entire process on track, long-range project planning is needed. Several meetings will need to be scheduled in advance, additional meetings may become necessary, meeting rooms of sufficient capacity will need to be booked, and materials will need to be produced for each meeting. Depending on the previous commitments and schedules of the involved stakeholders, planning and scheduling each meeting, one at a time, may result in considerable delays. Therefore, advanced planning is a very good idea and is typically dependent upon having administrative staff available to focus on this matter.

5. Determine a strategy for managing conflicts and reaching consensus

The process of reaching consensus about need priorities and related solutions involves managing disagreements and conflicts of interests. As individuals may have strongly held values about specific need areas of concern, meeting discussions can become more interesting than you may have anticipated. While it is important to let all participants get their views on the table, it is also important to keep blood off the table. That calls for a strategy and some skill in managing conflict and helping participants negotiate. It may be helpful to involve a facilitator or to discuss possible group decision-making strategies with individuals who have experience with similar group processes (see Chapter 6).

6. Determine a strategy for building ongoing coalitions

For decisions about need priorities and potentially workable solutions to be turned into enacted and funded programs and policies, coalitions will need to be fostered during the needs assessment process. The foundation for these coalitions will come from the stakeholders involved. Instead of waiting until the results are in and then looking to build the coalitions needed to give the final report political support, a coalition-building focus should be established and maintained throughout the process. Failure to build a coalition of interested groups and parties to spearhead the end stage of the process can render useless all the other efforts. Coalition building is a strategic objective of needs assessment processes and it needs a strategy (see Chapter 7).

Data Stage

The data stage mainly focuses on identifying the statistical indicators, data sources, and other information needed to carry out the needs analysis functions. This is the stage that is often initially visualized when one thinks of needs assessments. It entails two essential parts: (1) identifying what you want and (2) pulling it together in a useful format. The key steps and issues to be addressed in this stage are as follows.

1. Identify indicators to characterize need

The first step in the data stage is the identification of the need indicators that will be used in the needs assessment process. Those responsible for selecting the indicators should have already been identified, as should have the procedures they will use. Many public health fields have already developed extensive lists of need indicators and the U.S. 2010 National Health Objectives provides another listing for consideration (Pickin and St. Leger, 1993; Klerman et al., 1984; Maternal and Child Health Model Working Group, 1997; Family Health Outcomes Project, 1997; HSRA, 1999).

2. Identify available data sources

Once an initial list of need indicators has been established, attention can be directed at determining data sources available to calculate the selected need indicators for the target population. A variety of types of data sources may be considered, ranging from computerized databases on individuals to published reports containing aggregated data. As available data sources are identified, an appraisal should be made of the expertise that will be needed to use the data sources, e.g., individuals with statistical computing and computerized information management skills.

3. Identify other data needed and a strategy for obtaining them

Once the data sources available to the needs assessment effort have been catalogued, an appraisal of what data are not readily available needs to be made. The amount of time, personnel effort, and cost required to obtain these desired data should be taken in account. Some revision of the extent of data to be considered in the needs assessment process may be called for in order to keep the overall project within its budget and time limits. Finally, a detailed plan is needed to establish how, when, and by whom the data will be obtained. Funds and personnel will need to be allocated to the task, which might include contracting for the development of data collection instruments, designing and conducting surveys, and holding focus groups.

4. Identify data to create a Resource Inventory

Resource Inventories are used to describe current activities and providers (resources) in terms of their distribution, scope and scale of operations, content, accessibility, and availability (McKillip, 1987). Such inventories are employed to estimate the extent to which there are current resources available to meet identified needs and thereby determine the level and location of unmet needs. The inventory of services should extend beyond the operations of the programs administered by the agency conducting the needs assessment and should include other services and providers available for the target population. Stakeholders are often good sources of information about external resource capacity and can be effective in expanding the description of current service capacity in a geographic area.

5. Assemble data

Assemble the data—how simply stated; but, of course, it is not so easily done as said. It is not enough to calculate the values of the selected need indicators, by time period, by target population subgroup, and by geographic area. These data need to be organized and summarized in a format that can facilitate discussions of need priorities. The operational definitions of the indicators will need to be explained. Number-filled tables may need to be reduced to a figure or map. As many of the individuals involved in those discussions will not have backgrounds in public health statistics, the data need to be presented in such a way as to be useful for all participants. Dense reports containing seemingly endless tables do not facilitate discussion, although they are often useful background information and supporting references for those who want to see everything. Repeated attempts to reorganize and summarize the data may be needed to support needs analysis.

Needs Analysis Stage

In actuality, the major steps in needs analysis are not so much discrete steps as an iterative process. At this stage in the needs assessment, the emphasis is on decision-making and consensus building. While this stage focuses on reaching conclusions about need priorities and workable solutions, achieving these objectives entails managing disagreements about values and negotiating compromises in the face of political realities.

1. Prioritize needs in terms of importance

The process of ranking or prioritizing needs in terms of importance is the first step in the needs analysis stage. This activity involves reaching an agreement among the stakeholders about which needs are most important. This task will be dealt with in greater detail in Chapter 5. Arriving at a group consensus on need priorities is a major milestone in the needs assessment process. Taking time to celebrate this accomplishment with those involved is warranted and promotes the positive team spirit that will be needed to reach the next milestones.

2. Determine sub-populations to which specific needs apply

Not all of the identified needs apply to the entire target population. Identifying specific population subgroups, such as, teens, minorities, or the elderly, for which specific needs apply is an important step in targeting solutions and reaching agreements about distinctive solutions best suited to that population. Separating needs for prioritization by subpopulations is also an effective means of managing disagreement, as it circumvents the conflicts that may arise from pitting the interests of one population segment, e.g., children, against those of another, e.g., the elderly.

3. Identify workable solutions to address needs

For a list of needs to be useful to policymakers, potentially effective programmatic and policy solutions must be identified that are judged to be acceptable to the public and policymakers, taking into account cost, practicality, cultural sensitivity, and so on. Methods for identifying a range of possible workable solutions and organizing them by their unique approach to address needs is covered in detail in Chapter 6.

4. Reassess needs in light of available solutions

For some needs, a workable solution may not be evident after taking into account potential effectiveness, efficiency, and acceptability. This may call for a reassessment of need priorities to give greater preference for needs that are more amenable to improvement. This does not suggest that the importance of any need is diminished. Instead, it recognizes that, with limited resources available, some realignment of priorities may be needed to give greater weight to those needs for which there is the greatest chance for improvement. This step allows those involved in the process to reexamine their need ranking in light of these realities.

5. Identify available resources to meet needs

Once needs and solutions have been prioritized, the next step in the needs assessment process is a review of the public and private resources available for meeting needs. Through this review, which involves the examination of information collected into an inventory of resources, a determination can be made of what current services are already online to meet needs. This step is important to reduce program and policy proposals that might result in duplicated services and redundant policies. Moreover, it can provide recognition for what current providers are already doing, while reducing possible opposition from groups that might feel their operations will be threatened by new initiatives.

6. Reach consensus among stakeholders regarding priority unmet needs and best solutions for specific subpopulations

The last step in the needs analysis stage involves affirming the priority unmet needs of the target population, along with identifying the best workable solutions for addressing those needs. This is done using the appraisal of current service and resource availability. This task further involves identifying those subpopulations and geographic areas in which unmet needs are greatest and affirming that the proposed solutions are best suited to each distinct population subgroup. Reaching a consensus among the stakeholders on this final objective of the needs analysis stage is a momentous milestone. Again, celebration is required, not just because of the achievement. The team effort and collegiality that allowed for this accomplishment needs to be continued. Needs analysis is not the end point of needs assessment.

Program and Policy Development Stage

After spending considerable energy on needs analysis, this next stage is even more critical and energy intensive. These tasks require well-developed leadership skills in consensus building, negotiation, change management, communication, and advocacy.

1. Develop plans to translate need statements and related solutions into policy

Developing feasible strategies and action plans to translate need statements and related initiatives into programs and policy is an important step toward making change happen. Involving individuals who have well-developed skills in the political process is invaluable to the success of this endeavor. Involving some of those individuals from the very start of the needs assessment process is clearly a decided advantage.

2. Secure internal agency approval of policy action plans

Programs often need internal agency approval before undertaking efforts to effect policy initiatives. Before proceeding too far with the development of policy action plans, this check point must be passed. Again, the appropriate representatives should have been involved and informed from the start of the needs assessment process.

3. Communicate results of needs analysis and policy action plans to advocacy groups, the general public, and other agencies

Once a policy action plan is in place, it is time to disseminate the results of the needs analysis to the public, other agencies, policymakers, and advocacy groups. This is not the time for springing unpleasant surprises but instead is the time to use the disclosure of information to garner support for the policy action plan. Media consultants can assist in orchestrating the dissemination of the results in an effective manner. Moreover, the stakeholders who were involved in the process can play a key role in distributing the needs analysis results and laying the groundwork for a positive reception.

4. Collaborate and cooperate with advocacy groups and related agencies to foster support for program and policy proposals

Collaboration and cooperation are the key components of this vital step toward generating support and momentum for the policy action plan and its proposals. Just as the aggregating and analyzing of data for needs analysis called for expertise in biostatistics, this step calls for the ongoing involvement of specialists who can keep working with the partners who make up the coalition that will support the results of the needs assessment. Compromises may need to be made to keep the coalition together and viable. Leaving things to chance at this stage is in effect an abandonment of the process. Personnel must be identified to keep "working the system" and to assure those who were involved in the process up to this point that their investment of time and effort was valued and well-spent.

5. Develop plans for monitoring and evaluating your proposed programmatic and policy initiatives when implemented

Assuming success from the needs assessment process in terms of getting programmatic and policy initiatives approved and funded, these efforts need to be monitored and evaluated. The foundation for this should have begun as the initiatives were being developed. To ensure that there are adequate data to assess their effectiveness during the next needs assessment, monitoring systems for collecting program performance data need to be planned and implemented. Hence, the needs assessment cycle starts again.

Resource Allocation Stage

Another important stage in the total needs assessment process is the allocation of resources to communities to address their specific level and diversity of needs. The use of funding formulas has gathered increasing interest in public health as a means to provide a rational and objective basis for the equitable distribution of funds and other resources among geopolitical units. This important aspect of needs assessment will be covered in greater detail in Chapter 5.

Discussion Questions

1. Considering the states of Old Virginia and New Carolina, what are the benefits and disadvantages of beginning the needs assessment process with an internal analysis of existing data which is then brought to the public versus beginning with a solicitation of public input on needs which is then supplemented with existing data?

2. Considering the state of Central Dakota, what are the risks of ceding "control" of a public health needs assessment process to private concerns? Is it essential that core staff be part of the health department? What are the benefits of private sector interest in public health needs assessment?

3. Given the old adage "all politics are local," how much flexibility should be built in for local assessments within an overall statewide needs assessment effort? What are the benefits and risks of a more formally controlled process from the state level versus a looser process that allows for local discretion?

4. Assuming our premise that public input is essential, how might this best be accomplished? What are some strategies for encouraging public participation in this process? Assess and rate each of the three case examples on their likely success in securing meaningful public input into the needs assessments described.

5. What are the advantages and disadvantages of identifying target populations or target problems before initiating the needs assessment process, as in the case of Central Dakota?

3

Data Sources for Public Health Needs Assessment

Sources of Data

The word *data* is of Latin origin* and refers to a collection of facts that together provide information; this information in turn leads us to know, to reason, to discuss, and ultimately, to act. Data are critical to needs assessment, because without data our knowledge is founded on opinion and speculation, not on factual information. At the same time, public health professionals have a responsibility to gather both opinion and fact to render a reasoned judgment on the actual presence or absence of need. Actions taken in response to identified needs must meet community standards to be accepted and institutionalized. Facts alone are insufficient for successful action.

Public health professionals utilize a wide array of data for assessment, planning, policy development, program implementation, monitoring, and evaluation. These data are available in varying formats and from multiple sources. *Secondary data* refers to those data that have been already collected, usually for a different purpose, but are available for such things as needs assessments. Census data are an example of secondary data, already collected, but very useful for needs assessments. *Primary data* refers to those data collected directly for the express purposes for which they will be used. A random survey of homeless families designed to ascertain their needs for housing, health ser-

---

*Datum, from the Latin *dare*, to give. A thing given or granted; something known or assumed as fact and made the basis of reasoning or calculation; an assumption or premise from which inferences are drawn. *The Compact Edition of the Oxford English Dictionary*, 1971, Oxford University Press.

vices, food, and employment assistance is an example of primary data collected specifically for a needs assessment of homeless families.

Primary or secondary data sources can be characterized as quantitative or qualitative, a somewhat dubious distinction. Quantitative data are often viewed as objective, numeric data. Qualitative data are alternatively considered as subject and nonnumeric. In reality, qualitative data are often coded into numeric values and quantitative data may reflect subjective categories. Both can be assembled, summarized, analyzed, and used effectively to characterize needs in populations. For purposes of needs assessments, the types of data typically utilized can be categorized into four areas (population-based social indicator data, survey data, structured group data, and program-based data), each of which may contain elements of primary, secondary, quantitative, and qualitative data. Table 3.1 illustrates this, where two check marks indicate the more typical emphasis of each type of data and one check mark indicates a less typical emphasis.

In the process of assessing needs, public health agencies and professionals should optimize the data already available to them, if for no other reason than to avoid costly duplication of information already gathered. If available data have largely been identified and mined for information relevant to the needs assessment process and gaps still exist in our knowledge of needs, then some type of primary data collection is in order. Finally, it is often useful to use some form of primary data approach to help interpret the data that already exist, or that have been collected through a previous needs assessment process. Let us discuss each type of data and the sources that can be used by public health professionals for needs assessments.

Population-Based Social Indicator Data

This category of needs assessment data includes data collected by the Bureau of the Census and that collected as part of state vital record systems.

Table 3.1. Types of Data for Needs Assessments

Type of data for needs assessment	Primary	Secondary	Quantitative	Qualitative
Population-based social indicator data		✓✓	✓✓	
Survey data	✓✓	✓✓	✓✓	✓
Structured group data	✓✓	✓		✓✓
Program-based data		✓✓	✓✓	✓

Each of these meets the definition of "population-based" as these databases are intended to enumerate all events of interest, such as all births, all deaths, or all persons residing in a particular neighborhood. Census data are particularly important to public health as they provide critical denominator data in the calculation of rates. It is not enough to know that 200 persons died of a particular disease in a given community; we must also know how many people were potentially at risk for the disease. Was it 200 out of 200? That's a serious problem! Or was it 200 out of 2 million?

$$\text{Rate} = \frac{\text{\# of specified events}}{\text{\# of persons at risk for a specified period of time x constant (e.g., 1000)}}$$

Census data also provide public health professionals with a wealth of information on socioeconomic factors that can affect, positively or negatively, the health of people within given neighborhoods. Data on household size, housing quality, family income, age, and ethnic composition of neighborhoods provide important contextual variables in the interpretation of health data gathered through other avenues. Census data assist in the interpretation of health status and health risk indicators, of health resource access and utilization, and of community perceptions of health needs. Census data are available on the entire population at the level of the nation, individual states, and standard metropolitan statistical areas, right down to the level of individual "census tracts." Census data are also essential for mapping and generating visual displays of the sociodemographic characteristics of particular communities.

Vital record data include birth and death certificates, and records of marriages, divorces and adoptions. Vital record reporting is based on state law, not federal. Therefore, there are variations among states in certificates, reporting procedures, data availability and quality. Vital record data are population-based and contain data not only on the health or vital event itself (e.g., the birth or the death) but also on medical, health, and social factors potentially involved in the vital event. In these ways, vital record data provide an important and ongoing source of information on populations at particular periods of vulnerability; e.g., pregnancy and childbirth, and at the time of death. From vital record data are derived infant mortality rates, cause-specific mortality rates (e.g., deaths due to cardiac conditions, motor vehicle accidents or cancers) among many other statistical indicators of health. Table 3.2 provides a list of potential health status outcome and health risk indicators that can be created from birth certificate data.

Table 3.2. Possible Indicators from Birth Certificate Data

Mortality indicators	
Infant	Cause-specific
Postneonatal	Perinatal
Neonatal	SIDS
Hebdomadal	Injuries, firearms

Birth outcomes	
High birth weight	Low birth weight
Very low birth weight	Postterm
Preterm	Very preterm
Small for gestational age	Average for gestational age
Large for gestational age	

Socioeconomic risk factors	
Maternal age, young or old	Educational attainment
Urban/suburban/rural status	Parity
Interpregnancy interval	Race/ethnicity
Marital status	

Health care utilization	
Prenatal care	

Medical risk	
Poor previous pregnancy outcomes	Diabetes
Hypertension	Tobacco, alcohol, and drug use

While all states generally adhere to the standard certificates developed every 10 years by the National Center for Health Statistics of the U.S. Department of Health and Human Services, states can also choose to delete items or add items of particular relevance to their state or to collect data not routinely collected by other states. A draft copy of the upcoming (Year 2002) US standard birth certificate is displayed as Fig. 3.1 (NCHS, 2000).

One example of data not routinely collected by all states is reports of induced terminations of pregnancy; while all states report abortions, these data are collected in different ways, some on the individual level, others in the aggregate, so that the information is not necessarily comparable (CDC, 1999).

Population-based social indicator (census and vital record) data possess distinct strengths for purposes of needs assessments (McKillip, 1987):

- Data are available within broad geographic areas.
- Data are available on a large number of individuals or cases.
- Data are inexpensive to use.

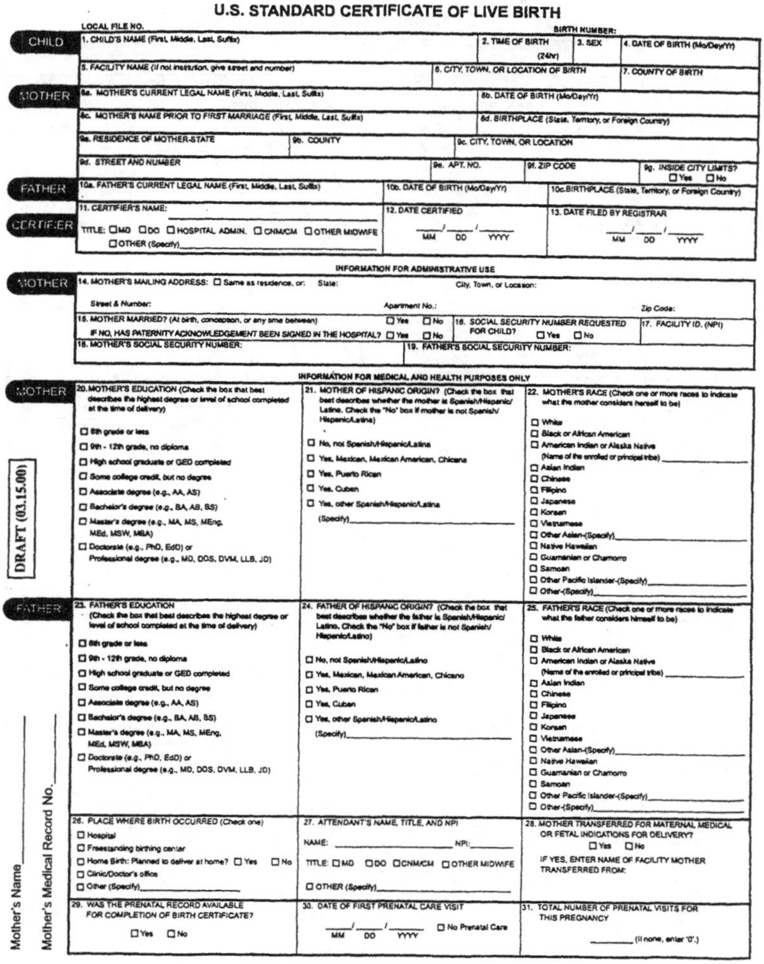

U.S. STANDARD CERTIFICATE OF LIVE BIRTH

LOCAL FILE NO.
BIRTH NUMBER:

CHILD
1. CHILD'S NAME (First, Middle, Last, Suffix)
2. TIME OF BIRTH (24hr)
3. SEX
4. DATE OF BIRTH (Mo/Day/Yr)
5. FACILITY NAME (If not institution, give street and number)
6. CITY, TOWN, OR LOCATION OF BIRTH
7. COUNTY OF BIRTH

MOTHER
8a. MOTHER'S CURRENT LEGAL NAME (First, Middle, Last, Suffix)
8b. DATE OF BIRTH (Mo/Day/Yr)
8c. MOTHER'S NAME PRIOR TO FIRST MARRIAGE (First, Middle, Last, Suffix)
8d. BIRTHPLACE (State, Territory, or Foreign Country)
9a. RESIDENCE OF MOTHER-STATE
9b. COUNTY
9c. CITY, TOWN, OR LOCATION
9d. STREET AND NUMBER
9e. APT. NO.
9f. ZIP CODE
9g. INSIDE CITY LIMITS? ☐ Yes ☐ No

FATHER
10a. FATHER'S CURRENT LEGAL NAME (First, Middle, Last, Suffix)
10b. DATE OF BIRTH (Mo/Day/Yr)
10c. BIRTHPLACE (State, Territory, or Foreign Country)

CERTIFIER
11. CERTIFIER'S NAME: ______
TITLE: ☐ MD ☐ DO ☐ HOSPITAL ADMIN. ☐ CNM/CM ☐ OTHER MIDWIFE
☐ OTHER (Specify) ______
12. DATE CERTIFIED ___/___/___ MM DD YYYY
13. DATE FILED BY REGISTRAR ___/___/___ MM DD YYYY

INFORMATION FOR ADMINISTRATIVE USE

MOTHER
14. MOTHER'S MAILING ADDRESS: ☐ Same as residence, or: State: City, Town, or Location:
Street & Number: Apartment No.: Zip Code:
15. MOTHER MARRIED? (At birth, conception, or any time between) ☐ Yes ☐ No
IF NO, HAS PATERNITY ACKNOWLEDGEMENT BEEN SIGNED IN THE HOSPITAL? ☐ Yes ☐ No
16. SOCIAL SECURITY NUMBER REQUESTED FOR CHILD? ☐ Yes ☐ No
17. FACILITY ID. (NPI)
18. MOTHER'S SOCIAL SECURITY NUMBER:
19. FATHER'S SOCIAL SECURITY NUMBER:

INFORMATION FOR MEDICAL AND HEALTH PURPOSES ONLY

MOTHER
20. MOTHER'S EDUCATION (Check the box that best describes the highest degree or level of school completed at the time of delivery)
☐ 8th grade or less
☐ 9th - 12th grade, no diploma
☐ High school graduate or GED completed
☐ Some college credit, but no degree
☐ Associate degree (e.g., AA, AS)
☐ Bachelor's degree (e.g., BA, AB, BS)
☐ Master's degree (e.g., MA, MS, MEng, MEd, MSW, MBA)
☐ Doctorate (e.g., PhD, EdD) or Professional degree (e.g., MD, DDS, DVM, LLB, JD)

21. MOTHER OF HISPANIC ORIGIN? (Check the box that best describes whether the mother is Spanish/Hispanic/Latina. Check the "No" box if mother is not Spanish/Hispanic/Latina)
☐ No, not Spanish/Hispanic/Latina
☐ Yes, Mexican, Mexican American, Chicana
☐ Yes, Puerto Rican
☐ Yes, Cuban
☐ Yes, other Spanish/Hispanic/Latina (Specify) ______

22. MOTHER'S RACE (Check one or more races to indicate what the mother considers herself to be)
☐ White
☐ Black or African American
☐ American Indian or Alaska Native (Name of the enrolled or principal tribe) ______
☐ Asian Indian
☐ Chinese
☐ Filipino
☐ Japanese
☐ Korean
☐ Vietnamese
☐ Other Asian-(Specify) ______
☐ Native Hawaiian
☐ Guamanian or Chamorro
☐ Samoan
☐ Other Pacific Islander-(Specify) ______
☐ Other-(Specify) ______

DRAFT (03.15.00)

FATHER
23. FATHER'S EDUCATION (Check the box that best describes the highest degree or level of school completed at the time of delivery)
☐ 8th grade or less
☐ 9th - 12th grade, no diploma
☐ High school graduate or GED completed
☐ Some college credit, but no degree
☐ Associate degree (e.g., AA, AS)
☐ Bachelor's degree (e.g., BA, AB, BS)
☐ Master's degree (e.g., MA, MS, MEng, MEd, MSW, MBA)
☐ Doctorate (e.g., PhD, EdD) or Professional degree (e.g., MD, DDS, DVM, LLB, JD)

24. FATHER OF HISPANIC ORIGIN? (Check the box that best describes whether the father is Spanish/Hispanic/Latino. Check the "No" box if father is not Spanish/Hispanic/Latino)
☐ No, not Spanish/Hispanic/Latino
☐ Yes, Mexican, Mexican American, Chicano
☐ Yes, Puerto Rican
☐ Yes, Cuban
☐ Yes, other Spanish/Hispanic/Latino (Specify) ______

25. FATHER'S RACE (Check one or more races to indicate what the father considers himself to be)
☐ White
☐ Black or African American
☐ American Indian or Alaska Native (Name of the enrolled or principal tribe) ______
☐ Asian Indian
☐ Chinese
☐ Filipino
☐ Japanese
☐ Korean
☐ Vietnamese
☐ Other Asian-(Specify) ______
☐ Native Hawaiian
☐ Guamanian or Chamorro
☐ Samoan
☐ Other Pacific Islander-(Specify) ______
☐ Other-(Specify) ______

26. PLACE WHERE BIRTH OCCURRED (Check one)
☐ Hospital
☐ Freestanding birthing center
☐ Home Birth: Planned to deliver at home? ☐ Yes ☐ No
☐ Clinic/Doctor's office
☐ Other (Specify) ______

27. ATTENDANT'S NAME, TITLE, AND NPI
NAME: ______ NPI: ______
TITLE: ☐ MD ☐ DO ☐ CNM/CM ☐ OTHER MIDWIFE
☐ OTHER (Specify) ______

28. MOTHER TRANSFERRED FOR MATERNAL MEDICAL OR FETAL INDICATIONS FOR DELIVERY? ☐ Yes ☐ No
IF YES, ENTER NAME OF FACILITY MOTHER TRANSFERRED FROM:

29. WAS THE PRENATAL RECORD AVAILABLE FOR COMPLETION OF BIRTH CERTIFICATE? ☐ Yes ☐ No

30. DATE OF FIRST PRENATAL CARE VISIT ___/___/___ MM DD YYYY ☐ No Prenatal Care

31. TOTAL NUMBER OF PRENATAL VISITS FOR THIS PREGNANCY ______ (If none, enter '0'.)

Mother's Name ______
Mother's Medical Record No. ______

Figure 3.1. Upcoming U.S. standard birth certificate.

U.S. STANDARD CERTIFICATE OF LIVE BIRTH

MOTHER

32. MOTHER'S HEIGHT ______ (inches)

33. MOTHER'S PREPREGNANCY WEIGHT (or weight at first prenatal visit) ______ (pounds)

34. MOTHER'S WEIGHT AT DELIVERY (or weight at last prenatal visit) ______ (pounds)

35. DID MOTHER GET WIC FOOD FOR HERSELF DURING THIS PREGNANCY? ☐ Yes ☐ No

36. NUMBER OF PREVIOUS LIVE BIRTHS (Do not include this child)
- 36a. Now Living — Number ______ ☐ None
- 36b. Now Dead — Number ______ ☐ None
- 36c. DATE OF LAST LIVE BIRTH ___/___ MM YYYY

37. NUMBER OF OTHER PREGNANCY OUTCOMES (spontaneous or induced losses or ectopic pregnancies)
- 37a. OTHER OUTCOMES — Number ______ ☐ None
- 37b. DATE OF LAST OTHER PREGNANCY OUTCOME ___/___ MM YYYY

38. CIGARETTE SMOKING BEFORE AND DURING PREGNANCY
Please answer for each time period.
(If none, enter "0". 1 pack = 20 cigarettes)
Average number of cigarettes smoked per day:
- Three Months Before Pregnancy ______
- First Three Months of Pregnancy ______
- Second Three Months of Pregnancy ______
- Last Three Months of Pregnancy ______

39. PRINCIPAL SOURCE OF PAYMENT FOR THIS DELIVERY
- ☐ Private Insurance
- ☐ Medicaid
- ☐ Self-pay
- ☐ Other (Specify) ______

40. DATE LAST NORMAL MENSES BEGAN ___/___/___ MM DD YYYY

41. MOTHER'S MEDICAL RECORD NUMBER

MEDICAL AND HEALTH INFORMATION

42. RISK FACTORS IN THIS PREGNANCY (Check all that apply):
- Diabetes
  - ☐ Prepregnancy (Diagnosis prior to this pregnancy)
  - ☐ Gestational (Diagnosis in this pregnancy)
- Hypertension
  - ☐ Prepregnancy (Chronic)
  - ☐ Gestational (PIH, preeclampsia, eclampsia)
- ☐ Previous preterm births
- ☐ Other previous poor pregnancy outcome (includes, perinatal death, small-for-gestational age/intrauterine growth restricted birth)
- ☐ Vaginal bleeding during this pregnancy prior to the onset of labor
- ☐ Pregnancy resulted from infertility treatment
- ☐ None of the above

43. INFECTIONS PRESENT AND/OR TREATED DURING THIS PREGANCY (Check all that apply):
- ☐ Gonorrhea
- ☐ Syphilis
- ☐ Herpes Simplex Virus (HSV)
- ☐ Chlamydia
- ☐ Hepatitis B
- ☐ Hepatitis C
- ☐ *None of the above*

44. OBSTETRIC PROCEDURES (Check all that apply)
- ☐ Cervical cerclage
- ☐ Tocolysis
- External cephalic version:
  - ☐ Successful
  - ☐ Failed
- ☐ None of the above

45. CHRONOLOGY OF LABOR AND DELIVERY
- A. Facility admission that included delivery ___/___/___ at ______ (MM DD YYYY, 24 hour clock) ☐ Delivery not in facility
- B. Rupture of membranes occurred on: ___/___/___ at ______ (MM DD YYYY, 24 hour clock) ☐ Not applicable ☐ Unknown date and time
- C. Onset of labor occurred on: ___/___/___ at ______ (MM DD YYYY, 24 hour clock) ☐ Not applicable ☐ Unknown date and time
- D. Full cervical dilation occurred on: ___/___/___ at ______ (MM DD YYYY, 24 hour clock) ☐ Not applicable ☐ Unknown date and time

46. CHARACTERISTICS OF LABOR AND DELIVERY
- Induction of labor ☐ Yes ☐ No
- Augmentation of labor ☐ Yes ☐ No
- Non-vertex presentation ☐ Yes ☐ No
- Steroids (glucocorticoids) for fetal lung maturation received by the mother prior to delivery ☐ Yes ☐ No
- Antibiotics received by the mother during labor ☐ Yes ☐ No
- Clinical chorioamnionitis diagnosed during labor or maternal temperature ≥38°C (100.4°F) ☐ Yes ☐ No
- Moderate/heavy meconium staining of the amniotic fluid ☐ Yes ☐ No
- Fetal intolerance of labor such that one or more of the following actions was taken: in-utero resuscitation measures, further fetal assessment, or operative delivery ☐ Yes ☐ No
- Epidural or spinal anesthesia during labor ☐ Yes ☐ No

47. METHOD OF DELIVERY
- A. Was delivery attempted with forceps and/or vacuum extraction?
  - Attempted Forceps ☐ Yes ☐ No
  - Attempted Vacuum ☐ Yes ☐ No
- B. Fetal presentation at birth
  - ☐ Cephalic
  - ☐ Breech
  - ☐ Other
- C. Final route and method of delivery (Check one)
  - Vaginal:
    - ☐ Spontaneous
    - ☐ Forceps
    - ☐ Vacuum
  - Or,
    - ☐ Cesarean
  - *If cesarean, was a trial of labor attempted?* ☐ Yes ☐ No
- D. Has the mother had a previous cesarean delivery?
  - ☐ Yes *If Yes, how many* ______
  - ☐ No

48. MATERNAL MORBIDITY (Check all that apply) (occurring 24 hours before delivery or within 24 hours of delivery)
- ☐ Maternal transfusion
- ☐ Third or fourth degree perineal laceration
- ☐ Ruptured uterus
- ☐ Unplanned hysterectomy
- ☐ Admission to intensive care unit
- ☐ Unplanned operating room procedure following delivery
- ☐ None of the above

DRAFT (03.15.00)

NEWBORN INFORMATION

49. NEWBORN MEDICAL RECORD NUMBER:

50. BIRTHWEIGHT: ______ (grams)

51. OBSTETRIC ESTIMATE OF GESTATION: ______ (completed weeks)

52. APGAR SCORE:
- Score at 5 minutes: ______
- If 5 minute score is less than 6,
- Score at 10 minutes: ______

53. PLURALITY - Single, Twin, Triplet, etc. (Specify)

54. IF NOT SINGLE BIRTH - Born First, Second, Third, etc. (Specify)

55. ABNORMAL CONDITIONS OF THE NEWBORN (Occurring within 24 hours of delivery)
- Assisted ventilation required immediately following delivery ☐ Yes ☐ No
- Assisted ventilation required for more than six hours ☐ Yes ☐ No
- NICU admission ☐ Yes ☐ No
- Newborn given surfactant replacement therapy ☐ Yes ☐ No
- Antibiotics received by the newborn for suspected neonatal sepsis ☐ Yes ☐ No
- Seizure or serious neurologic dysfunction ☐ Yes ☐ No
- Significant birth injury (skeletal fracture(s), peripheral nerve injury, soft tissue or solid organ hemorrhage which requires intervention) ☐ Yes ☐ No
- If yes, (Specify) ______

56. CONGENITAL ANOMALIES OF THE NEWBORN (Check all that apply) (Observed within 24 hours of delivery)
- ☐ Neural tube defect
- ☐ Cyanotic congenital heart disease
- ☐ Congenital diaphragmatic hernia
- Anterior abdominal wall defect
  - ☐ Omphalocele
  - ☐ Gastroschisis
- ☐ Limb reduction defect (excluding congenital amputation and dwarfing syndromes)
- ☐ Orofacial defect/cleft
- ☐ Suspected chromosomal disorder
  - Karyotype confirmed ☐ Yes ☐ No
  - Karyotype pending ☐ Yes ☐ No
- ☐ Hypospadias
- ☐ None of the anomalies listed above

57. WAS INFANT TRANSFERRED WITHIN 24 HOURS OF DELIVERY? ☐ Yes ☐ No
IF YES, NAME OF FACILITY INFANT TRANSFERRED TO:

58. IS INFANT LIVING AT TIME OF REPORT? ☐ Yes ☐ No ☐ Transferred

59. IS INFANT BEING BREASTFED? ☐ Yes ☐ No

Mother's Name ______

Mother's Medical Record No. ______

Figure 3.1. (Continued)

- Data allow for entire populations to be described.
- Data are perceived as quantitative, credible and therefore also perceived as unbiased.
- Data are relatively easy to access.
- Data are available over time, so that trends can be analyzed.

Despite the relative strengths of these population-based social indicator databases, they also have inherent weaknesses:

- Any individual item may be of questionable validity.
- These data sets tend to reveal problems more readily than they do solutions.
- Specific variables of interest may not be included in these data sets.
- Because they are well established, it is difficult to alter the type of data collected.
- The data are not always available in a timely manner.

So, for instance, if one were interested in assessing trends in motor vehicle-related fatalities, one could use the U.S. death file to identify those deaths due to motor vehicle-related events. Such data could be examined in many ways to examine variations in trends in geographic regions of the country, among different age, race, and gender groups, and over time. However, if one were interested in nonfatal injuries or in the response time between the actual incident and the arrival of any emergency response personnel, those data would not be available on this file. Such an assessment would have to be conducted using other data sources, or perhaps by reviewing hospital discharge and emergency room data or by conducting record audits or surveys. Birth certificate data have been used for many years to examine the relationship between the initiation and number of prenatal care visits and the outcome of pregnancy; however, those data provide little to no information on the content of prenatal care. What actually takes place in an individual visit or over the course of a pregnancy must be ascertained through other data-gathering mechanisms such as medical chart reviews, surveys, or interviews of clients and providers.

Survey Data

Much of our knowledge about health status, the incidence of disease, and the presence of risk factors whether environmental, physical, or behavioral, is derived from surveys or surveillance systems. Surveillance is an essential component of public health practice and entails the detection, description, and geographic and temporal monitoring of health status problems and their determinants. The basic elements of surveillance include the *ongoing* and *systematic*:

- Collection of data
- Evaluation, consolidation, analysis, and interpretation of data
- Prompt dissemination of the synthesized results to the public, relevant stakeholders and decision/policymakers

Every state public health agency operates surveillance systems, typically in the area of communicable disease, but increasingly in the area of chronic disease. All states operate disease reporting systems; others have developed sophisticated registries of cancer cases or of birth defects. Environmental health programs also engage in surveillance of air, water, and food supplies to ensure their safety. Licensure and certification units monitor the quality of institutions, such as nursing homes, the credentials of health care providers, and hospital discharge data systems. As health care delivery systems have become more formally organized through various forms of managed care, health plans are developing what could be considered surveillance systems to monitor the attributes of their enrollees, the quality of care delivered, and the costs and health outcomes associated with that care. Unlike the public health sector, however, private health plans have no responsibility to release these data to the public.

Renewed interest in surveillance has arisen in the wake of growing concern over the possibility of bioterrorist attacks on U.S. targets. Bioterrorists use chemical or biologic agents to cause disease and death on a wide scale. A small amount of a biologic agent such as anthrax or smallpox released into the air or placed in a food or water supply can infect many people before the "attack" is ever recognized, creating wide-scale panic and resulting in the loss of many lives. On May 18, 1998, President Clinton issued Presidential Decision Directive 62, ordering federal agencies to take significantly expanded and better coordinated steps to protect against the consequence of biologic attacks, particularly those directed at civilian populations. A key component of this directive is the improvement of the nation's public health surveillance system so as to increase the ability to detect quickly, based on the appearance of specific disease symptoms, the presence of a biologic agent. The focus on such a system will have the added benefit of improving the reporting of diseases and disease precursors for other surveillance purposes, thereby providing more complete and accurate data for needs assessments.

If conducted periodically, surveys are a form of surveillance. Examples of national surveys that function in this way are the Behavioral Risk Factor Surveillance System and the Youth Risk Behavior Survey, and the National Health Interview Survey. Single, one-time surveys can also be used to answer a particular series of questions. The 1988 National Maternal and Infant Health Survey (NMIHS) and the 1991 Longitudinal Follow-up to the NMIHS are relevant examples of one-time national surveys, although the need for a repeat of the NMIHS continues to be a topic of discussion among public health advocates. Surveys are an important tool by which public health professionals gather and assess health status, health outcomes, risk exposure, and disease determinants among groups of people within various communities. Surveys can be used to gather and assess the opinions of stakeholders (those who have vested interests in either the process or the outcome of your needs assessment activities), as well as the opinions of the target population regarding perceived health status and health care needs. Further, surveys can be used to assess the perceived availability and scope of services as well as the level of utilization of health and related services within specified communities or among particular population groups.

As a powerful tool for gathering precise data on populations, issues, and variables of interest and of controversy, surveys are clearly an important and indispensable part of public health needs assessments. Surveys provide several important strengths (McKillip, 1987):

- Surveys allow for *direct feedback* to stakeholders and the public.
- Surveys can foster *public awareness* about a particular problem or area of concern.
- Surveys can be tailor-made to address specific issues.
- Surveys can be targeted to specific population groups or geographic areas.
- Surveys can provide very timely results.

As a note of caution, the development, administration, data analysis, and interpretation of surveys are very complex, requiring highly skilled, professionally trained individuals to ensure the integrity of survey data. The inherent weaknesses of surveys include:

- Surveys can be quite costly in addition to their complexity.
- Surveys require technological expertise to ensure the reliability and validity of the data.
- Surveys may not be representative or generalizable to other populations.
- Survey responses may reflect desires and not actual needs.
- Conducting surveys may arouse expectations that you may be unable to meet.
- Without careful quality controls, survey questions may reflect the biases of those who frame them.

As is the case with population-based social indicator data, much data have already been collected through national, state, local, or private surveys and may be available for you to use in your needs assessment efforts. More than 70 agencies of the federal government collect data and produce statistics of interest to public health professionals and the general public. These include such widely recognized surveys as the National Health Interview Survey, the National Health and Nutrition Examination Survey, the National Survey of Family Growth, and the National Electronic Injury Surveillance System (see Table 3.3). This list also includes surveys less familiar to the public such as the Pregnancy Risk Assessment Monitoring System, the Survey of Program Participation, the National Hospital Discharge Survey, and the Current Medicare Beneficiary Survey. The Federal Interagency Council on Statistical Policy maintains a Web site that provides easy access to the full range of data collected and produced by the U.S. federal government. This site can be accessed at http://www.fedstats.gov. Finally, surveys not necessarily considered in the public health arena are also conducted and may provide essential information to public health professionals. These include surveys conducted by news organizations, polling firms, and private foundations like the Pew Charitable Trusts, the Kaiser Family Foundation, and others.

Anyone can be surveyed: clients or consumers of services; key informants or community leaders; health and related service providers; employers and purchasers of health care; or members of the community or the population at large. As is the case with any data-gathering effort for the purposes of assessing needs, existing surveys should be identified and mined for all relevant information before a new survey is developed. At the same time, data gathered through established surveys should be thoroughly assessed for their relevance to the needs assessment task at hand, for their ability to provide detailed analysis in small geographic areas or within population subgroups, and for the extent of the population covered by the survey. For example, although Public Law 101-354, The Breast and Cervical Cancer Mortality Prevention Act of 1950, established the Surveillance, Epidemiology and End Results (SEER) program, not all states participate. As such, only participating states can accurately report the incidence of breast cancer and the nationwide incidence can only be estimated.

In spite of the availability of the results of numerous national and state surveys that have already been conducted, it is not unusual to find that the information wanted for a needs assessment is still unobtainable from current sources of data. This may result from several possible causes. First, the specific information desired may not have been collected on the original data sources. Such information may include details about your target population's

Table 3.3. **Examples of National Surveys and Surveillance Systems: United States, 1999**

Survey or surveillance system	Responsible agency
Medical Expenditure Panel Survey Healthcare Costs and Utilization Project Consumer Assessment of Health Plans	Agency for Healthcare Research and Quality (formerly the Agency for Health Care Policy and Research)
Behavioral Risk Factor Surveillance System Youth Risk Behavior Survey National Notifiable Diseases Surveillance System National Electronic Injury Surveillance System National Health and Nutrition Examination Survey	Centers for Disease Control and Prevention
National Health Interview Survey National Longitudinal Survey of Youth National Hospital Discharge Survey National Maternal and Infant Health Survey National Survey of Family Growth	National Center for Health Statistics
Toxic Releases Inventory Pollutant Release and Transfer Registers	Environmental Protection Agency
Uniform Crime Reports	Federal Bureau of Investigation
National Crime Victimization Survey	Department of Justice
Medicaid National Summary Statistics Medicaid Managed Care Enrollment Report Medicaid and Medicare Survey and Certification	Health Care Financing Administration

health-related behaviors and attitudes, perceptions of their own health status, feelings and beliefs about local priority needs, or opinions about their health care providers and system. Next, the available surveys that have collected the desired information may not be representative of the target population. Nationally representative surveys may have sampling designs that preclude making generalizations about subpopulations or specific geographic areas. Surveys from other states or regions may not reflect the circumstances or opinions of the target population in another state or region. Even a representative survey of a state may not provide a valid, generalizable sample of each locality or ethnic group within the state. The use of survey data that are not representative of the target population may be misleading to the needs assessment process or may generate dissension about the validity of the data and its interpretation. Accordingly, collecting primary data to inform the needs assessment may become necessary and will often be heartily endorsed by those involved in the needs assessment process. To ensure the success of the needs assessment activity in reaching a consensus about needs and related policy and program solutions, collecting primary data may be unavoidable and beneficial, if it can be done within time and cost limitations.

Several issues should be carefully reviewed when making decisions about collecting primary data for a needs assessment. While it would be ideal to have information from all members of the target population, carrying out a full census is simply unrealistic in most cases due to the expense. The next alternative to a census is a survey, which entails impartially collecting timely information from a representative sample of the target population in a manner that is systematic, standardized, and replicable. While far less expensive than a full census, surveys are still expensive and time-consuming and require expertise. A brief review of the steps in designing a survey will quickly reveal why the decision to undertake a survey should be made only after a careful consideration of all that is involved.

There are a number of important questions to resolve in designing a survey. First, the purpose of the survey needs to be explicitly established. If information is only needed for a specific point in time, then a one-time survey will suffice. If trend data are needed, then multiple surveys may be necessary. The precise information to be obtained through the survey must be clearly spelled out and the specific questions to be asked must be delineated. Once the decision is made to conduct a survey, there may be a natural tendency to add additional questions to the original list of needed items (i.e., since we have already gone to the trouble of getting them to answer a few questions, couldn't we ask them just a few more?). Accordingly, the questions to be queried can quickly grow in number. As they do, it may become more difficult to keep a focus on what is essential and how the growing amount of information will be effectively used to identify, prioritize, and address unmet need areas. It should also be pointed out that an agency and human subjects panel review and approval of the survey plan, the data collection instrument, and the informed consent form may likely be required before the survey can be conducted.

To ensure the generalizability of a survey, a representative sample will need to be drawn. The selection of a sample entails the consideration of statistical issues and it is highly advisable that appropriate expertise be involved in developing the sampling frame and in determining how many individuals should be surveyed. Next, a survey method will need to be chosen. Possible surveying approaches include face-to-face or telephone interviews and mailed (or even Internet) questionnaires. For whatever approach is selected, the survey collection tool, e.g., the mailed questionnaire or the interview guide, will need to be developed, formatted, and pretested. Interviewers may need to be trained. Finally, the information collected on the survey form will need to be coded, entered for computer analysis, cleaned, analyzed, and prepared into reports for interpretation and use. Refused, incomplete, and missing responses must also be assessed. From the development and administration of surveys through the statistical analysis and interpretation of their results, consultation and involvement from suitably trained and experienced experts are needed.

Given what is entailed in planning and conducting a valid, representative survey, it is not surprising that successfully carrying out a survey that accomplishes its purpose is expensive and time-consuming. In order to save some money, the scope of a survey can be pared down to the most essential elements, although the need (and cost) for expert involvement in the survey remains. Unfortunately, the more circumscribed objectives of a Spartan survey may raise questions about whether the very limited information obtained is worth the cost or, if implemented, may only lead to the demand for more detailed information. These many practical concerns about undertaking any survey may lead to looking for yet another more cost-effective approach to collecting primary data. That alternative is the small or structured group study, which, like the survey, allows for the collection of primary data and further allows for acquiring much more extensive information. But, while gathering information from a small study group is far more economical than surveying a population sample, the information derived from a small group may not in any way reflect or be representative of the opinions and circumstances of the entire population. Ideally, having both representative survey data and in-depth small group data can provide a rich resource of information. However, cost and time restraints often necessitate making difficult choices and having to settle with what is less than ideal. The particulars of structured small group data will be addressed in the next section.

Structured Group Data

Unlike population-based data systems, surveillance networks, or surveys that gather data from individuals, structured group data are derived from formal or informal gatherings of individuals, for the purpose of assessing the interactions among the participants and gauging the opinions of the entire group. Structured groups generally fall into two categories: those that are assembled very purposefully, such as focus groups or advisory panels, or those that are loosely convened, such as public hearings or town forums.

Structured groups provide qualitative data that can be very useful in designing quantitative data collection systems by suggesting reasonable and appropriate avenues of enquiry or in identifying the potential content of population or opinion surveys; in gathering data that are difficult to obtain through quantitative methods; or in interpreting the results of other quantitative data gathering efforts. Structured groups provide the means for various stakeholders to define what they believe to be their needs in terms of those things they either desire or expect from their community, the health care system, or public agencies. These group members can confirm the situation revealed by population-based social indicator data, or that obtained through surveys, or their observations can enhance the information gleaned from these data. They can elucidate the factors potentially underlying findings from other data collection systems. And, they can identify issues perceived by the participants as important that may not have been considered by program personnel or policymakers.

Structured groups have many strengths (McKillip, 1987):

- Structured groups involve people from the target audience, key informants, stakeholders, and the general community in direct conversation about possible health needs.
- Structured groups can foster acceptance for the entire needs assessment process within the community and various target populations.
- Structured groups provide the means to tap into perceptions, opinions,

and desires of people in ways that no other data collection methodology can.

- Structured groups can generate new ideas about problems that exist as well as potential solutions.
- Structured groups can be conducted relatively quickly providing immediate feedback to program planners, evaluators, or policymakers.
- Structured groups are relatively inexpensive compared to other methods of needs assessment data collection.

At the same time, structured groups present several weaknesses that must be considered when utilizing them in needs assessment efforts:

- Structured groups suffer from the bias introduced by lack of representativeness. The convener of a structured group may have little control over who chooses to attend and participate.
- Related to the first weakness, structured groups may be dominated by outspoken members whose opinions may not reflect those of the larger group.
- Further, structured groups do not provide the investigator with any consensus on an issue. Even if everyone in the group agrees, because they may not represent the views of the larger community, such broad consensus cannot be construed.
- While structured groups are useful for introducing the needs assessment and planning process to the community, such activities also build expectations. "You asked my opinion and I gave it to you, but you ignored it—nothing has changed."
- It is difficult, but possible, to convert the results of structured group assessments into a quantifiable form, i.e., into numbers, percentages, or rates.

Perhaps the most familiar form of structured group is the *focus group*. It is critical to note here that the focus group is a technique that, if used correctly, can yield important insights into the perceptions and opinions of a target population. Unfortunately, the term is often misused—throwing people together into a room and asking them a few questions does not a focus group make! Similar to surveys, it is preferable to engage someone with expertise in the design and conduct of focus groups to ensure the usefulness of their results.

Some critical factors in successful focus groups will be noted here. Readers interested in more detail on this subject are directed to an excellent text by Richard A. Krueger, *Focus Groups: A Practical Guide for Applied Research* (Sage Publications, 1994).

Focus groups provide a forum for focused discussion on the topic or topics of interest to you in your needs assessment efforts. You will be assembling groups of people to respond to, and discuss as a group, a series of questions. This discussion will be guided by a facilitator. You will need to work hard to design a set of questions that elicit the information you are seeking without suggesting that there is a "right" or "wrong" answer to the questions. The questions must engender discussion among the group to be of most value to you. Remember that the focus group is a data-gathering tool, one of several you will be using in your needs assessment process. You are not asking the advice of the participants nor are you seeking consensus. You simply want to know what they think about a particular topic or series of related topics. The role of the facilitator is critical in focus groups and if you have the resources, you may wish to engage a professional facilitator. The facilitator must be skilled in keeping the conversation balanced—drawing out participants who are quieter and politely subduing those who tend to dominate the conversation. A good facilitator will also follow-up on interesting comments, even if they deviate slightly from the question being asked. To free the facilitator to truly facilitate, you will also need a recorder, someone who is not part of the discussion but who is taking notes, audiotaping or in some cases videotaping the discussion. Recording aids in later transcription, but remember, you must always seek permission to record a focus group.

To be most informative, you need to conduct a series of focus groups in order to detect trends across members of your target population. Remember that any one group can be dominated by an outspoken member or may, for whatever reason, have little to say or have opinions far removed from those of the general populace. Each group must be of a size large enough to generate discussion but small enough so that every member has the opportunity to participate (6 to 10 is considered the appropriate size of any individual group). While the collective of focus groups you assemble should be reasonably representative of the entire target population, each individual focus group should be as homogeneous as possible and the individual participants unknown to each other. This homogeneity and unfamiliarity are both critical to eliciting open and frank discussion. People are more comfortable in a room of people who are similar to them, be it in age, gender, socioeconomic status, culture, or ethnicity, and will feel freer to express their opinions. However, if they know other persons in the room, they may be more reticent in their comments.

Seeking to understand the reasons women do or do not seek and obtain routine prenatal care during pregnancy, the Maryland Healthy Mothers, Healthy Babies Coalition convened a series of focus groups across the state. Each group was comprised of a relatively homogeneous group, but collectively, these focus groups yielded critical information from low-income, rural, teenaged, urban, middle-to-upper income, and older women, military dependents, couples, and reproductive health care providers.

Also useful in gathering public input on an issue are so-called town meetings or public forums at which interested members of the community are invited to speak, often for a set number of minutes, to express their opinions on the issue being discussed. These hearings are typically posted in newspapers or community newsletters and are at a date and time convenient for members of the community to participate. Depending on the nature of the issue, or the level of anticipated controversy, they may be broadcast over other media (radio or television) or covered by news media outlets. Whether or not to widen a highway; whether or not to allow a variance in zoning requirements for a particular property; whether or not to locate a waste site in a neighborhood; whether or not to install traffic signals at a particular intersection; whether or not to allow a group home for recovering alcoholics/victims of domestic abuse/runaway teenagers/the mentally ill or developmentally disabled in a particular neighborhood; these are all examples of the types of issues that may be addressed at a public hearing or town meeting. Local community groups or advocacy organizations may promote attendance at such hearings and may produce written testimony for the record. They may arrange transportation and provide informational materials describing their point of view. Communities across the globe use the town meeting both to impart information and to gather opinions. In the late 1990s in the United States, President Clinton successfully used the town meeting to speak directly with interested citizens on topics of interest to his administration, including such things as health care reform, race relations, and violent crime.

Service and Program Data

Most, if not all, public health programs operated by public sector agencies maintain databases necessary for the effective management of the program. These databases are often a rich source of data useful for needs assessments in that they contain comprehensive data on clients served, dollars spent, activities undertaken, and results achieved for critical public health efforts. Many of these databases provide good information on expressed needs, i.e., services utilized as an expression of demand, while others may provide population-level data on disease incidence, provider and facility utilization, provider availability, or costs associated with particular services. These databases associated with programs and services are not found exclusively within public health agencies or health departments. Databases of interest to public health practitioners seeking to identify health needs or emerging health trends may be found in environmental management agencies, education departments, human service agencies, corrections and criminal apprehension agencies, and other publicly funded organizations serving citizens. The data maintained by private sector health plans on providers, clients, claims, and quality assurance activities may also be important sources of data for needs assessment as are those maintained by state Medicaid agencies.

Providing important data on expressed need or demands for service, service and program databases can provide a wealth of information on defined sets of clients and on specific types of services. Those databases that serve as management information systems for client-serving programs can provide data on the utilization of services including information on the recipients of services, the providers of services, the nature and scope of services received, costs of services, and referrals to other service providers. Depending on the sophistication of the database, it may contain case management data or data on the outcomes or results of services and recommendations for services needed in the future. Programs that serve communities rather than individual clients also maintain databases important to public health needs assessments. Data on food, water, and air quality monitoring, applications for and renewals of certain professional licenses, records of violations, or incidents of noncompliance with certain regulations may facilitate understanding of both health status indicators and the possible factors that underlie their geographic variation. With regard to program management, service and program databases are invaluable for monitoring and evaluating the success of the program in meeting its stated objectives as well as assessing the fiscal efficiency with which the program was run. These data are often helpful in documenting the ongoing need for the program and for the allocation of continuing or additional resources. It is important to note, however, that service and program databases do not reflect communitywide needs and their exclusive use may preclude consideration of alternative solutions to the problems already identified. While useful to document the need for programs in terms of demand, they are not sufficient to determine the effectiveness or efficiency of programs, nor whether needs have been met or remain unmet. Importantly, program data cannot speak to the needs of those who do not use the program's services, whether eligible for them or not.

Service and program databases possess many strengths promoting their use as one component of a comprehensive needs assessment:

- They typically have been in existence for quite some time and so contain data collected over many years.
- The data within these databases are usually housed on-site and are readily accessible by existing program staff.
- As such, these data can be readily accessed, and because they are typically very current, they provide the most timely data of all data sources.
- As the databases already exist, they are relatively inexpensive to operate and to maintain. Creating service and program databases can be relatively expensive, but once they exist, the annualized costs can be fairly well controlled.

As indicated earlier, service and program databases suffer from some inherent weaknesses that must be considered when these data are utilized for needs assessment purposes:

- Service and program databases do not provide data on unmet needs not addressed by the program or service.
- Service and program databases address demand for only those programs or services.
- Service and program databases do not provide data that are representative of the total target population, only on those who seek and receive the service or program.
- Though designed for managerial and administrative purposes, some of the data elements contained in service and program databases may be of uncertain quality.

Registries are the exception to these caveats in that when well designed, these program databases can capture close to 100% of the events of interest. At the federal level, the Centers for Disease Control and Prevention operate the

National Notifiable Diseases Surveillance System, to which states report 60 infectious diseases, as a means of tracking the incidence, prevalence, and survival rate of specific reportable diseases. In addition to infectious diseases, many states operate registries to track chronic diseases such as cancer and traumatic brain and spinal cord injuries; the incidence of birth defects and congenital anomalies; and, in recent years, immunizations. These registries not only serve to track the incidence of particular diseases and associated risk factors but to allow for the assessment of the effectiveness of various interventions. Like other aspects of public health surveillance, the requirements for notifiable diseases (i.e., those diseases that health care providers, laboratories, and other health professionals are required to report to state health departments) are legislated and/or regulated by individual states (CDC, 2000). To improve the comparability of disease reporting across states, the Centers for Disease Control and Prevention in conjunction with the association of state epidemiologists, developed a set of Case Definitions for Public Health Surveillance (CDC, 1990). The CDC Surveillance Group also develops case definitions for a broad range of noninfectious diseases, including injuries, occupational or environmental conditions, chronic diseases, and adverse reproductive health events (CDC, 2000).

Private Sector Data

Increasingly, due to health reform and cost containment efforts or market-driven changes in the health care delivery and financing systems, state public health agencies are asked to contribute to policy debates that demand high quality information on which to base decisions. In their evaluation of the Robert Wood Johnson Foundation's Information for State Health Policy Program, Feldman and colleagues noted that while many state health databases are technically sophisticated, they are strategically weak, meaning that the data that are available are not necessarily helpful in formulating effective policy (Feldman et al., 1994). Fortunately or unfortunately, many public health databases are funded, and their design directed, by federal agencies. This has undoubtedly facilitated the development of health-oriented data systems and strengthened the quality of data in programs across the country. At the same time, this activist federal role may have inadvertently driven states to adopt a passive role in the development of data systems that can also contribute to state program and policy development activities.

On the positive front, the growth in managed care and in competition among health plans has stimulated the development of standard "report cards," the most famous of which is the Health Plan Employer Data and Information Set (HEDIS), which consists of a standardized set of performance measures in quality of health care, access to care, patient satisfaction, membership in the plan, utilization of services, and financial issues (NCQA, 1996). While this movement has increased the ability of employers and purchasers, consumers, regulators, and advocates to compare performance across health plans, this data set still does not provide population-based data and so is less powerful for community-level needs assessment efforts.

Public health professionals engaging in needs assessments must always be mindful of those data elements that are *not* available on secondary data sets and must consider whether or not their absence warrants primary data collection. Considerations of cost, timing, and benefits of investing in primary data collection are helpful in determining an appropriate course of action.

Discussion Questions

1. Given the topics of interest to the private sector in the state of Central Dakota (i.e., adolescent pregnancy, domestic violence, and workplace injuries), for each one, please consider sources of data. Include population, survey, structured group, and program database sources. Which are more likely to require primary data collection? Which strategies of primary data collection might you employ for those that require the gathering of new information?

2. Design a strategy for using focus groups in a local community to assess needs for the following potential public heath initiatives:
   • Improving the breast-feeding rate
   • Improving early detection of colorectal cancer
   • Decreasing the incidence of sexually transmitted diseases
   • Promoting access to dental care for children and the elderly

3. Review the Year 2002 US Standard Certificate of Live Birth included in this chapter. Consider items to be used for purposes of ongoing needs assessment around the health of women of reproductive age that you believe should have been included that are not.

4. Your county is experiencing repeated violations of the Environmental Protection Agency's standards for tropospheric ozone and you are under the
   gun to develop a long-term solution to this problem. You know it is essential to assess the public's understanding of the problem, their perception of
   its importance, and their willingness to accept any solution you might im-
   pose. You are considering such interventions as cleaner but more expensive
   gasoline, mandatory vehicle emissions testing, and the development of mass
   transit systems. Please consider the advantages and disadvantages of using
   a survey versus a structured group approach for gathering this information
   from the members of your community.

5. The public has told you that they are concerned about what appears to be a
   growing number of injuries in the state. Other than mortality data, you have
   no statewide system for monitoring injury occurrence. You have identified
   a number of program specific databases that include information on injuries from such disparate sources as the Emergency Medical System, Law
   Enforcement Crime and Victim Reports, the Department of Boating and
   Recreation, the Regional Burn Center, and the School Violence Prevention
   Initiative. First, consider the likely content and quality of each of these
   databases. Next, consider the credibility of each in the mind of the public
   and decision-makers. What strategies will you use to compile, weigh, interpret, and apply these data to enhance your understanding of the nature and
   extent of the problem of injury morbidity in your state?

4

Communicating Needs
for Community Action

The Critical Import of Communication

Needs assessment in public health is ultimately a public and political activity. The outputs of needs assessment will direct programmatic efforts, policies, and resources toward those conditions deemed to be of greatest public health importance and of greatest interest to the community. However, it sometimes happens that these two interests collide. That is, what the data suggest are the issues of greatest public health importance may be of little interest to the community, while an issue that engenders popular interest is not supported by the scientific knowledge-base or by the expert opinions of public health professionals. Despite this potential for conflict, thorough and successful needs assessment efforts strive to balance effectively data-based evidence with community sentiment and develop plans that are achievable in the pursuit of shared public health goals.

Essential to achieving this balance of scientific evidence and public comment, is communication. As such, communication, social marketing, and health education professionals are as important to successful needs assessments as are data analysts and research scientists. Communicating with the target audience for needs assessment, whether it be a focused constituency (e.g., adolescents or the elderly) or an entire community, is critical throughout the process. Accordingly, several basic tenets can be proposed to enhance communication:

- The target audience must be informed about the needs assessment process in its earliest stages and informed that a public health plan will be developed or modified to address current trends.

- The target audience must be given ample opportunity to contribute to all phases of the process, including the design, implementation, interpretation, and dissemination of the needs analysis.
- The target audience should have ample input into the establishment of need priorities and the development of the plan resulting from the needs assessment as programs, policies, and resources will be directed based on the results of the analysis.
- Finally, the target audience should be a critical partner in the ongoing monitoring of the identified health conditions of concern, the implementation of the plan, and the evaluation of the overall effort.

All this is to say that the community, or the target audience for the needs assessment and the subsequent plan must become *engaged in the process* from inception to conclusion and beyond. After all, needs assessment is a cyclic process including periodic assessments, ongoing health surveillance, monitoring of programmatic efficiency, evaluation of programmatic effectiveness, and reassessment of program and funding priorities. Because public health efforts are designed for the public, public input is critical to ensuring the best possible outcomes with the most efficient use of resources.

Steering Committees

One fairly simple way to promote communication with partner organizations and constituency groups is to establish a needs assessment steering committee. Such a committee would be charged with the responsibility of providing overarching guidance to the needs assessment effort; ensuring and creating opportunities for public input; and communicating with others outside the immediate group involved in the process. Each of these tasks is critical and together they suggest the types of persons you can and should invite to serve on the steering committee. Steering committees can also be subdivided into task-focused committees (e.g., data gathering and analysis, community involvement, partnerships), allowing for more members and optimizing people's talents where they will be best utilized. Possible members of a steering committee for public health needs assessment efforts include:

- Community organizations or advocacy groups interested in the issue(s) to be addressed through the needs assessment

- Key leaders in the community, including business, church, and community members perceived as leaders in the community
- Consumers or recipients of services associated with the topics being addressed
- Providers of services associated with the topics being addressed
- Representatives of "sister" agencies (depending on how the state or community is organized and the focus of the needs assessment effort, you may wish to involve representatives of agencies responsible for the environment, welfare or social services, health insurance or Medicaid, education, commerce, community development, or transportation)
- Researchers or academicians with expertise in the areas to be addressed

Because the steering committee can be subdivided into committees, the overall steering committee itself should be convened early in the process and maintained throughout the needs assessment cycle. Despite the time invested in convening, staffing, and utilizing a steering committee, effective steering committees will pay dividends far beyond the initial investment. Steering committees not only provide valuable guidance and direction, the members serve as critical information and communication conduits to their specific constituencies helping maintain awareness of the process as it unfolds and facilitating mutual understanding of the desires of the agency conducting the assessment and the wishes of the public. Steering committees also promote visibility of your efforts in the broad community. Steering committees can hold hearings or town meetings as described in Chapter 3, which in turn become communication vehicles in and of themselves. Steering committee meetings on special topics may even capture the attention of the media, generating further awareness and interest in your efforts.

Communicating through Data Gathering

As discussed in Chapter 3, the act of gathering primary data is in and of itself a form of communication to the public, the target audience, or a constituency group for your needs assessment efforts. By surveying, interviewing, or assembling members of your constituency into groups for the express purpose of soliciting opinions, you are informing them of your activities, your areas of interest, and in some cases, the directions you may be considering. Key informant interviews are a critical means of both gathering important information from and communicating information to a specific target community. While steering committee members can help serve this purpose, there will always be other knowledgeable members of the community with whom you will wish to discuss your needs assessment efforts. Depending on your focus, you will want to consider meeting with leaders of coalitions, community groups, and citizens organizations concerned with the topic of your assessment. Business and community leaders, elected politicians, judges, religious leaders, and neighborhood activists are all potential sources of information for *you* about the community and for the *community* about you.

Conducting surveys or focus groups or convening town meetings will also educate and inform members of the target population about your efforts while allowing you to gather much-needed data on the subject matter of interest. Market researchers will tell you that engaging in product research will generate interest in a product, sometimes enthusiastic, sometimes negative. Not everyone will support the approach you are taking, your needs assessment activities, or even your agency. Your gathering data and asking questions may alarm some people, raise their anxiety, or be threatening to them. An extreme example of this is in the area of substance-abusing pregnant women. In the late 1980s and early 1990s, several states added the reporting of alcohol or substance use during pregnancy to the birth certificate and others enacted legislation requiring health care providers to screen and report pregnant or postpartum women found to be using or abusing drugs. While the intent was ostensibly to ensure access to needed services for the mother, and to ensure the interests of the child were protected, such legislation had the chilling effect of frightening pregnant women away from the prenatal health care system. The desire to better quantify the extent of alcohol and substance use during pregnancy and the presence of such substances in newborns may have forced some pregnant women to go underground, thereby precluding not only valid data collection but more importantly, the provision of appropriate and necessary services (Connolly and Marshall, 1991; Moseley and Bell, 1991)

Media Partnerships

While many people are loathe to appear on television or to be interviewed by the press, the media (television, radio, and print) provide powerful communication tools for public health needs assessment efforts. Indeed, over the next few days, start reading your daily newspaper with an eye toward health-related articles. We guarantee you will find something every day. Whether it's a report from prestigious medical journals like the *New England Journal of Medicine* or the *Journal of the American Medical Association*, the latest survey results on the health behaviors of Americans (or the residents of your state or local community), a human interest story about a person or family who has survived a debilitating illness, or the latest diet or exercise fad, you will find articles that provide health information, statistical facts, or perspectives on health status, health risks, longevity, and quality of life. Be assured, if there is a report on a hazardous chemical emanating from a nearby factory, pollution in the air or water, or the dangers of imported vegetables, as a public health professional, you had best be prepared to respond to the concerns such a report will generate among the public. Whether or not these issues emerged from your internal analyses of your sources of data, they will be on the public's mind.

Despite what public health practitioners might feel on any given day, the public is interested in health in general, and is particularly interested in threats to their health. Moreover, the public wants to know ways to promote their health and that of their families and the communities in which they live. Many Americans take for granted that the water is always safe, that a meal at a restaurant won't kill them, that they are safe at their place of work, and that their children will not be exposed to toxic substances at the local playground. In fact, public health agencies are constantly working behind the scenes to ensure that these beliefs are upheld and that public health systems do not fail. Media provides an important vehicle to communicate both health information and the public health agency's role in gathering and disseminating that information.

You can utilize the print media in several ways. Foremost in this area is contributing a press release or a letter to the editor on your launching of a comprehensive needs assessment effort. Providing a review of what is known about a particular public health issue, or a commentary on an issue that has been previously covered by the media is another means of engaging the media in the needs assessment process. Working with a reporter to prepare a report on your activities often starts by issuing an invitation to attend a town meeting or forum or focus group on your needs assessment (see Chapter 3 for a discussion of structured groups as a source of data for needs assessments), or by arranging to be interviewed on a subject relevant to the needs assessment process (the issuing of a data report, an innovative strategy to obtain public input, the development of health objectives for the community, an evaluation of a program in your agency).

Television and radio are also important sources for health information.

These media outlets are required by the Federal Communications Commission to provide a certain number of hours of public health service air time, free of charge each day. Many public health agencies have developed public service announcements or have worked in partnership with other interested organizations to purchase air time for important public health messages. So effective can these messages be, that the requirement that antitobacco messages be given equal air time to protobacco messages led to the tobacco industry's voluntary cessation of television and radio tobacco advertising in the mid 1960s (U.S. Department of Health and Human Services, 1989). Short of free public service announcements, radio and television media are also powerful communication vehicles and can be utilized just as the print media to help inform the public about your efforts and your message. Most local markets sponsor local news or talk shows that are usually happy to cover events of local interest; to interview you for a story relevant to your efforts; or to feature some aspect of your overall effort to help engage the public in the debate you are encouraging.

Media personnel may also call you, often unexpectedly, and want you to appear on a show, or be interviewed for a story. Some tips to keep in mind when responding to this type of media invitation:

- Always *request the questions ahead of time* so you can prepare responses—if they won't give them to you, you can respectfully decline the interview.
- Regardless of the questions they intend to ask you, prepare *three points* that you want to make sure you get across in the interview (the audience may remember three points, they will not remember more); you have certainly noticed how people savvy with the media will not really answer the question, but will make their own points over and over again.
- If you will be including any data in your responses, *keep them very simple* and make sure the numbers enhance your points, not detract from them.
- Finally, most public agencies have a media relations person and protocol regarding media contacts. Always clear any media contact with the appropriate person before responding.

Clearly, media promotions of health messages are an important part of the overall public health strategy to promote and protect health. Such messages can also be helpful in promoting the needs assessment concept and encouraging citizens to participate. Public health agencies can issue press releases, hold press conferences, or simply advertise upcoming events. Data on particular topics can be released to the media, as can the results of a survey or series of focus groups (the annual release of birth and infant mortality statistics is usually covered by the media). The media can announce a town meeting or can solicit public comment on a report or draft strategic plan. Particularly at the local level, news media outlets in small- and medium-sized cities or towns are often eager for stories of local interest and are happy to promote participation in community needs assessments. Of course, nothing engenders public interest like controversy and the media often play a pivotal role in the outcome of a needs assessment process by expressing editorial opinions about a particular problem or solution, publishing arguments from opposing sides on a controversial issue, or objectively covering the events as they unfold. In these ways, public opinion is informed and positions taken; once again, communication of the facts, the alternatives, and the consequences of different courses of action becomes very important to ensure open debate and agreement on the ultimate solutions. Chapters 5 and 6 continue this discussion in greater detail by addressing methods for establishing priorities and selecting feasible solutions to identified public health problems.

Communicating Data

Communicating data can be a tricky undertaking. While on the one hand, data must be provided within their appropriate context and with complete information to facilitate their interpretation, on the other hand, data should be provided in a manner that allows the reader to quickly grasp the message and should not be so detailed that they are uninterpretable to the lay public. As endless data tables and sophisticated statistical analyses are not the stuff of quick study, simple, understandable statistical indicators have been developed and the public has become accustomed to them. The birth rate, the infant mortality rate, the adolescent pregnancy rate, the motor vehicle death rate, the cancer incidence rate, the unemployment rate, the high school graduation rate, the rate of injuries to certain classes of workers, the crime rate, these are all facts and figures with which the public is generally familiar and that can be quickly grasped and understood. Something is getting better, something is getting worse. These are powerful communication tools that can greatly assist in engaging the public and soliciting their opinions about these and other health conditions. Unfortunately, there are many areas of concern to the public for which no statistical indicator is available; there are some for which no data-base is readily accessible or even in existence. For these, we must utilize other methods of assessing health status, identifying threats or risks to health, and eliciting the concerns of the public. (See Chapter 3 for an in-depth discussion of the various sources of data used in public health needs assessments.)

Graphical displays of data rather than tabulations of numbers are gener-ally more effective in communicating data-based messages. Consider the ex-amples shown in Table 4.1 (good presentation of information) and Figure 4.1 (better presentation), and again in Table 4.2 (good presentation) and Figure 4.2 (better). Notice how much more easily you grasp the message in the charts than you do in the tables, even though the information presented is identical.

Communicating through Technology

Increasingly, in this era of rapidly advancing computer technology, fed-eral, state, and local health agencies are developing Web sites that are easily

Table 4.1. Preterm Birth, Inadequate Prenatal Care Use and Neonatal Mortality: 1981–1996 Live Births to U.S. Resident Mothers

Year	Very low birth weight	Very preterm	Low birth weight	Preterm	Neonatal mortality	% inadequate prenatal care	% intensive prenatal care	Infant mortality
1981	1.16	1.81	6.8	9.4	8	13.5	3.4	11.9
1982	1.18	1.84	6.8	9.5	7.7	13.6	3.6	11.5
1983	1.19	1.86	6.8	9.6	7.3	12.9	3.9	11.2
1984	1.19	1.83	6.7	9.4	7	12.7	4	10.8
1985	1.21	1.88	6.8	10	7	12.4	4.4	10.6
1986	1.21	1.9	6.8	10.2	6.7	12.1	4.9	10.4
1987	1.24	1.96	6.9	10.2	6.5	11.8	5.3	10.1
1988	1.24	1.96	6.9	10.6	6.2	11.9	5.4	10
1989	1.28	1.95	7	10.6	5.8	12.5	5.9	9.2
1990	1.27	1.92	7	10.8	5.8	12.1	5.9	9.2
1991	1.29	1.94	7.1	10.7	5.6	11.6	5.9	8.9
1992	1.29	1.91	7.1	11	5.4	10.9	6.1	8.5
1993	1.33	1.93	7.2	11	5.3	10	6.3	8.4
1994	1.33	1.89	7.3	11	5.1	9.4	6.4	8
1995	1.35	1.89	7.3	11	4.9	9	6.7	7.6
1996	1.37	1.89	7.4	11	4.8			7.3

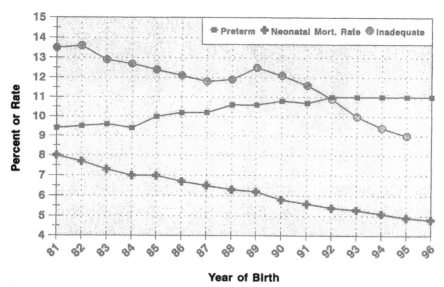

Year of Birth

Figure 4.1. Preterm birth, inadequate prenatal care use, and neonatal mortality: 1981–1996 live births to U.S. resident mothers.

accessed by the public, other providers, and interested community organizations. Some areas have developed particularly innovative uses of the Internet for communicating health information, soliciting ideas and comments from constituent groups, and for informing the community about needs assessments, program innovations, or related events. It is conceivable that you could develop a Web page exclusively for the purposes of your needs assessment effort.

Technical reports developed as part of the needs assessment process are

Table 4.2. Proportion of Total Annual Deaths by Cause of Death Nonwhite Males, 15–19 Years of Age

Cause of death	Proportion of total annual deaths
Drowning	7%
Stabbing	8%
Motor vehicle	19%
Firearm	33%
Other injury	9%
Noninjury	25%
Total	100%

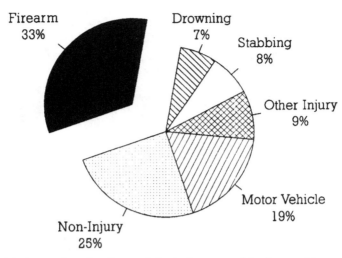

Figure 4.2. Proportion of total annual deaths by cause of death: nonwhite males, 15–19 years of age.

often very useful documents . . . unfortunately, they are not always dissemi-nated to the right people, and not everyone has the inclination or the time to wade through them. Even more frustrating is learning that such a report exists and then being unable to access a copy. Placing these reports on a Web site gives them a longer "shelf life" and draws attention to them. Providing the executive summary and key conclusions on a Web page makes it easy for inter-ested persons to quickly grasp the essence of the report.

Communicating in the Legislative Arena

Ultimately, it is in the legislative arena that the voice of the public is heard most resoundingly. Unless you have the luxury of modifying the direction of a particular program or shifting resources from one area of interest to another within the purview of your internal programmatic responsibility, you will have to present any recommendations for change in policy, programmatic effort, or direction or allocation of resources to decision-making bodies outside your agency. Typically within state government, such programmatic initiatives must first pass internal muster and then must be reviewed and approved by staff of the governor's office, including those with responsibilities for fiscal, legal, human resource, and political affairs. If your initiative is approved at this level, it can be presented to the legislature as part of a governor's package. The governor may not oppose your effort but may not include it in his or her package; in this case, you may be free to take it to the legislature directly. If rejected completely, you may still be able to gain a legislative audience through the efforts of advocacy or community groups. Obviously, in any case, the knowledgeable support of the community for whom the policy or programmatic effort is designed will be critical to your success in the legislative arena.

In addition to offering testimony on a particular piece of legislation or appropriations bill (always consistent with the position of your agency and the governor's office), you may be invited or have the opportunity to speak at a legislative hearing around a particular topic to which no actual piece of legislation is attached. Members of legislative committees, special commissions, or blue ribbon panels often hold hearings simply to gather information and opinion or to discuss possible legislative proposals around a topic of interest. These provide a nice opportunity for you to inform not only members of the legislature about your efforts but members of the public as well. Members of the public are often in attendance at these hearings, which are often reported by the media. Chapter 7 provides greater detail on the legislative process and how to achieve success in carrying out the directives of a needs assessment.

The public can influence the legislative process in many different ways. Legislators are people like the rest of us and usually have a group of trusted friends who they rely on to advise them on various pieces of legislation or appropriations bills. They also respond to the recommendations of professional groups with whom they have developed good relationships. Constituents may call, write, e-mail, petition, or visit their representatives expressing their opinion (usually strongly worded!) for or against a particular initiative. If strong public opinion is being expressed on a particular issue, the media will usually weigh in, giving credence to or disparaging a particular point of view. Finally, the public can and will make its feelings known at scheduled hearings on particular pieces of legislation, perhaps through organized demonstrations, by crowding the hearing room or by testifying on the merits or flaws of the proposal.

If you have never been to a legislative hearing at the state level, or a council hearing at the local level, or even a congressional hearing at the federal level, you must make a point of attending. The authors of this textbook have experienced hundreds of motorcycle enthusiasts on Harley Davidsons circling the state capitol during a hearing on whether or not to require motorcyclists to wear helmets (the bill was defeated); dozens of children with severe handicaps in a state capitol hearing room when a proposal to reduce spending for home-based services was being considered (the funds were restored); and one lone father with a baby walking the halls of the state capitol advocating for a bill requiring certain tests be performed prior to postpartum hospital discharge to prevent the illness that killed his wife (the bill was passed). Never underestimate the power of the public to influence the legislative process. Effective communication on your part throughout the needs assessment process can mobilize a group of constituents in support of the efforts you jointly conceive and develop. It also can stave off uninformed criticism of these efforts or can redirect energies from a less effective to a more effective solution.

Critical Partnerships

Ultimately, your success will depend on your ability to effectively communicate both *the needs* and your *plans to address the needs* to those in a position to approve and support your efforts. Translating the data gathered through this process into a plan of action that is acceptable to the public, to decision-makers,and to policymakers, and is ultimately funded, is the goal of needs assessment and depends on the effectiveness with which you communicate with and motivate others to work with you. As in all human interrelationships, there either has to be a common goal toward which different people are working, or an expectation that efforts made today will be rewarded tomorrow, the famous "quid pro quo." In Chapter 7 we discuss coalition building and the importance of involving a broad base of constituencies in your efforts. Remember though that if others have helped you secure the necessary support for your programs, they will expect you either to continue to involve them in some way, or to help them when they are in a situation of similarly needing external affirmation of their plans and proposals. Like all other aspects of needs assessment, this one is cyclic too, in that the communication about efforts and the willingness to work with others to get the job done, are never-ending.

Public health professionals are often heard bemoaning the fact that they typically have far fewer resources to share than do other agencies or private institutions. They feel that they cannot be equal partners in these joint ventures because they have no money to put on the table. We couldn't disagree more. Because of its population and community focus, public health often brings to the table what no one else can: population-based data and full knowledge of health status, health care utilization patterns, health system attributes, and broad demographic and community factors that impact nearly every intervention directed at people. Public health data provide critical denominators for the calculation of rates and for planning the scope of programmatic interventions. The broad knowledge of the community is also linked to public health's prevention focus, typically lacking in other organizations whose mission it is to treat apparent problems. Public health also brings a network of local contacts, across a state or across a county, that can be mobilized for various tasks, be they educational, data gathering, or direct interventions.

Discussion Questions

1. The Commissioner of Health for the state of Central Dakota is going to suggest to the two health plans that have come to enlist her assistance in their efforts, that a steering committee be established for this purpose. The commissioner intends to present a completed plan for the health plans' consideration, rather than asking them to identify the people who should serve on the steering committee. She has asked you to develop this plan for her review. Who do you believe should serve on this steering committee? Should there be subcommittees recommended at this time? If yes, who should serve on these?

2. Review the case example for the state of New Carolina. What would be the advantages and disadvantages of assembling a *state level* "assessment committee"?

3. The state of Old Virginia has presented its five year public health plan to the legislature, distributed the plan to local health officials at the state's annual public health conference, and placed the plan on the Internet to promote public access. What other means of communication could the state health department have used to promote this plan?

4. You've been called by a local newspaper reporter who has discovered that the state health agency distributed a pamphlet entitled "How to Use a Condom" at the recent state education conference. The reporter wants to interview you on the agency's rationale for promoting sexual behavior among

young people. How will you respond? (Will you answer his questions on the spot? Are there any data you might like to share with the reporter? What key points do you want to make in this interview?)

5. Several recent outbreaks of food-borne illness have alarmed the public, and in response community leaders are calling for action to make sure the food supply remains safe. Who would you like to have working with you on a Food Safety Coalition? Remember to think broadly.

6. Many groups outside the health department conduct needs assessments on populations and on health-related topics similar to those of interest to public health, e.g., hospitals, health plans, schools, private voluntary and nonprofit organizations. How can you develop sustained, ongoing relationships with these other organizations to assure better coordination and strategic planning, while understanding and respecting the independent missions of your and these other agencies?

5

The Selection and Use of Indicators

Statistical indicators of health status, health care utilization, health system attributes, and sociodemographic, economic, and medical risk are invaluable throughout the needs assessment process. As stressed earlier, statistical indicators facilitate comparisons among population subgroups, across geographic areas, and over time periods. Moreover, they aid not only in identifying problems and needs areas, but also in tracking and evaluating program performance and in allocating resources based on need and performance.

In this chapter, the selection and use of statistical indicators will be addressed from a number of perspectives. First, we will consider general criteria for selecting and assessing the utility of an indicator for needs analysis, performance measurement, and resource allocation. Moreover, we will explore possible techniques for establishing needs priorities. Next, our attention will turn to the consideration of additional criteria for selecting indicators for performance measurement. Finally, the use of indicators for resource allocation and for the development of funding formulas will be covered.

Indicator Selection Criteria

A substantial number of statistical indicators could potentially be proposed for inclusion in a comprehensive needs assessment. Indeed, with the growing proliferation of databases being employed in the health care field, it is likely that the number of indicators for which there is readily available data will continue to increase. However, finite resources for needs assessment activities preclude collecting data on every proposed indicator and this growing wealth of potential indicators may prove to be a pitfall. In addition to the expense involved in data collection, the inclusion of too many indicators may thwart a thoughtful and in-depth assessment and eventually overwhelm the process of establishing need priorities. Therefore, a clear plan is needed for selecting a manageable number of indicators that are individually distinct, accurately and systematically recorded, and relevant to the needs of the target population.

To keep the data collection stage of the needs assessment process workable, potential need indicators should first be organized by common or similar themes, such as, general disease type, environmental exposures, or injuries. Because many indicators address similar underlying health concerns, it is not necessary to collect data on every indicator related to that problem. For example, very low birth weight and preterm rates reflect similar perinatal problems and typically provide corresponding results, which in turn often concur with indicators of neonatal mortality and neonatal intensive care use. Therefore, by identifying the general health status concerns of interest in advance, e.g., perinatal outcomes related to prematurity at birth, it may be possible to focus on a single or more restricted number of representative indicators that will still reflect the overall health status of concern and be acceptable to the stakeholders involved in the needs assessment process.

As it is simply impractical to collect information on all possible indicators, the number of indicators for which data will collected must be reduced. Accordingly, criteria are needed to select those indicators that are perceived as the most useful. Data collection efforts would then be focused on those indicators that best meet the criteria and are not duplicative of others. The following criteria have been proposed for use in identifying indicators for needs assessment and surveillance efforts (U.S. Department of Health and Human Services, 1982; Hulsey, 1986). While this list represents the desirable attributes of indicators most useful for these purposes, it is recognized that few indicators are likely to meet all of these criteria. Hence, these criteria serve as a benchmark for weighing the potential costs and benefits of selecting one indicator over another.

- *Simplicity*. An indicator should be conceptually straightforward, well defined, reliable, and valid. It should be understandable to both the public and policymakers.
- *Stability*. Indicators should represent events with sufficient occurrence to provide stable estimates, i.e., estimates without dramatic fluctuation due to small numbers. Only in special cases, e.g., indicators of diseases with a high risk of spread or of death that are clearly preventable, should an indicator of an event with infrequent occurrence be used.

- *Availability.* The data needed to calculate the indicator should be timely and readily available, preferably at local, state, and national levels. This gives preference to indicators derived from data systems that are ongoing and updated frequently. Further, the cost of accessing or acquiring information must be economically feasible. To avoid having the needs assessment limited solely to those indicators contained on currently available databases, the prudent application of this criterion is encouraged. Establishing an ongoing survey or surveillance capacity is a long-term solution for increasing the availability of a wide array of need indicators.
- *Logical, Relevant, and Important.* An indicator should reflect the health status conditions and health system attributes it is intended to measure (concept validity). It should fall within the mission and goals of the agency and the objectives of relevant programs and policies. Further, a health status indicator should reflect sentinel and important public health concerns as indicated by their frequency, severity, and potential for spread or economic loss. Population and health care service indicators should reflect conditions and service patterns believed to be associated with changes in the health status outcomes of interest (predictive validity).
- *Broad Representation.* An indicator should reflect the potential health status concerns of the majority of the target population throughout the geopolitical subdivisions of the area served, as well as those of specific high-risk groups. The availability of a norm for comparisons is a positive attribute of an indicator.
- *Political Feasibility.* The selection of specific indicators should entail a consideration of the political climate and its relevance for intervention. However, this must be tempered by the potential impact of the problem on the public's overall health.

Establishing Need Priorities

A comprehensive needs assessment involves the consideration of diverse types of data, often of variable quality, derived from numerous sources by way of multiple data collection methods. Further, it entails the synthesis and interpretation of these data, taking into account the disparate and potentially conflicting value systems of the stakeholders. Once again, the core of needs assessment is not merely identifying needs and problems and linking them to solutions, but also achieving consensus among the stakeholders to support translating need statements into approved and funded program and policy initiatives. As needs assessment is a political act, the lack of sufficient consensus about the process or the findings may result in failure. It is during the initial process of establishing need priorities that the needs assessment process will face its first test with regard to consensus building.

No single strategy exists for successful consensus building but several skill areas are needed. Team building throughout the needs assessment process is of particular importance and must start early. Building a team requires leadership skills in building trust. Trust in the process is engendered by establishing and adhering to some basic principles about fairness, openness, and respect for the opinions of others. Team building also requires having a vision, a clear purpose, a plan to achieve that purpose, and the will to carry it through. As conflicts in values will arise in the needs assessment process, a strategy for conflict management will also be needed and should be thought through before the conflicts emerge. The team can be used to develop a means for addressing disagreements, and the successful resolution of initial conflicts may serve as an effective means of coalescing the group. Finally, as the data are many and the time is limited, meeting management skills are critical. Meetings are for making decisions and sharing opinions and information. Effective agendas specifically delineate the topic and time for each. Successful meetings emphasize decision-making.

Several strategies have been proposed for helping groups reach consensus about needs and establishing need priorities. One approach is to ask the participants in the needs assessment effort to give each need area a numeric rank score. Ranking is a process that encourages individual stakeholders to develop their own ranked priority list of need problem areas for the target population. Individual listings of ranked needs are then summed to create a composite or summary ranking. For example, participants might be asked to consider a tabulation of a diverse selection of need indicators for the population, e.g., rates of smoking by adolescents, motor vehicle deaths, mental disorders, dental caries, or infant mortality. These tables might further include some comparative rate information for other populations of interest, e.g., the total United States, the previous year or decade, or the surrounding region. Participants would then be asked to provide a numeric rank score for each need area ranging from "1" for the most pressing to the least pressing need. These scores would then be tabulated for all participants and a summary ranking produced. The ranges of the rankings for each needs area could also be examined to reveal consensus among the group.

Some discussion of the possible criteria for establishing a ranked priority score for each need area should be encouraged before the ranking process begins. Although individual values will play a role in determining the rankings, regardless of the criteria proposed, establishing general guidelines for setting priorities may aid in dealing with conflicting opinions and keep discussions focused. At a minimum, the ranking of need priority should consider: (1) the size of the problem (e.g., how many and what proportion of the population is affected by the problem) and (2) the seriousness of the problem, e.g., the severity in terms of health status (i.e., risk of mortality, morbidity, and long-term disability), economic loss to individuals and the community (including cost of care and loss of potential revenue), and the potential for spread or repeat of the problem (i.e., highly infectious or injurious conditions). Later in the process, attention will be given to whether there is an available solution to these identified problems. However, at this initial stage of identifying needs, it is enough to rank the needs in terms of importance without also focusing on the availability of effective solutions.

Reaching a final consensus on the list of ranked need priorities is often an iterative process. Before a final ranking of needs is established, individual rankings can be shared and discussed. Participants in the process should be encouraged to indicate why and how they arrived at the ranking. Once ample (but not unlimited) time has been given to this discussion, participants can be given the chance to change their rankings. A summary ranking can then be recalculated. Typically, no more than three renditions of this process should be needed to reach a fairly good consensus. This basic iterative process is sometimes referred to as Delphi approach.

The fundamental weakness of the ranking methodology for establishing need priorities is that it pits the needs of specific special interests groups against each other. For example, the needs of children become pitted against the needs of women, the environment against immunizations, injuries against chronic disease. Stakeholders may find it difficult to choose and conflicts may be difficult to resolve, even when using criteria that emphasize size and severity of the problem. The wider the scope of the agency, and the associated needs assessment effort, the larger this problem becomes. But even focused programs may have difficulties. One means of addressing this issue is to segment, or subdivide, target populations or general need areas prior to ranking to ensure that the needs of specific target population subgroups, e.g., infants, teens, adults, women, elderly, and children with special health care needs, are addressed. Need rankings can then be developed for each subpopulation. This approach of setting separate lists of need priorities can also be used for program topic areas, e.g., the environment, injuries, home health, genetics, maternity, and the like. The caveat to this approach is that it can be taken too far and eventually defeat the initial goal of establishing a list of need priorities.

Performance Measurement and Indicators

With passage in 1993 of Public Law 103-62 (the Government Performance and Results Act) and the movement of the federal Department of Health and Human Services toward performance partnerships in the early 1990s, the desire for greater accountability in publicly funded programs has flourished and performance measurement has become a required aspect of many federally funded program operations. Performance measurement is a natural outgrowth and component of a comprehensive needs assessment. In addition to meeting demands for accountability, it is part of the ongoing public health assessment function. By establishing performance benchmarks, public health programs can monitor and evaluate their progress toward addressing identified need areas. Further, once performance measurement and monitoring have become established, the next logical step will likely be the use of performance as the basis for funding and resource allocation to states and, in turn, localities.

The process of selecting performance measures should be integrated into established needs assessment activities. Similar to the determination of need indicators, the selection of performance indicators is also in part a political process, wherein consensus building is critical. Because many activities needed to reduce health status performance outcomes occur at the local level, collaboration between the state and local agencies is essential. To the extent that state funding may in the future reflect state performance and state funding is used to fund localities, state and local performance become inextricably linked.

Performance measures should be based on previously determined need priorities linked to specific solutions that fall under established public health approaches, e.g., direct services, enabling services, population-based services, and infrastructure building. Depending on the approach chosen, activities may be directed toward building capacity, undertaking processes, or reducing risk factors (Peoples-Sheps *et al.*, 1998). Performance measures quantify whether: (1) the capacity was actually built or strengthened, (2) the process or intervention was actually carried out, (3) the incidence of risk factors was reduced, and (4) health status was improved. In essence, performance indicators should measure any observable change from a previous state or level, which reflects the intended impact (or lack thereof) on program or policy action. These are the measures on which a program is willing to stake its worth and be judged. While the level of underimmunization of a population is a good indicator of need, the indicator of performance should reflect the level of change achieved in immunization rates, not simply the absence of need.

The criteria for selecting performance measures are similar to those proposed for need indicators (i.e., simplicity, stability, availability, logical, and broad representation). Several additional criteria for selecting performance measures have been proposed by the MCH Bureau in its Block Grant Guidance materials (HRSA, 1999). These are as follows:

- The measure is relevant to major state Title V activities and block grant dollars.
- The measure is applicable for the vast majority of states.
- The measure should be important and understandable to policymakers and the public.
- There should be a demonstrated link between the performance measure and the desired outcome.
- Data should be generally available from all states and jurisdictions.
- Measurable change in the performance measure should be expected within five years.
- If not a health outcome, the process or capacity building measure should clearly lead to an improved health outcome.
- Consideration should be given to the magnitude and feasibility of correcting the problem related to the performance measure, i.e., is the proposed change in the performance indicator realistic.
- The measure should be prevention focused.

The criterion for selecting performance measures that can be expected to improve within a five-year period deserves added emphasis. To follow this rule, health outcome performance measures should be limited to measures for which (1) the etiology or determinants of the outcome are well established and (2) there is a proven method for reducing the outcome incidence or prevalence. Similarly, performance measures of service utilization should be limited to measures for which (1) the determinants of utilization are well established and

(2) there are proven methods and adequate resources for reducing barriers to utilization, improving access, and extending outreach. While selecting only performance goals for which there is a logical approach to effect change may seem obvious, numerous performance measures have been proposed at both the state and national level that fail to meet these conditions. As such, it is highly unlikely that the performance will improve. This lack of improved performance will in turn beg explanations. To avoid a cycle of wishful speculations and fanciful conjectures about future and past performance, performance measures should remain grounded by existing evidence and avoid unrealistic aims, regardless of how popular.

Many of the indicators commonly used in needs assessments may not meet these additional requirements of having a clear etiology and an established method to effect change in the near future. This underlies an important difference between need and performance indicators and highlights that they are not interchangeable. In such cases where these added criteria are not met, those need indicators may make good monitoring measures, but poor performance measures. Good health outcome monitoring measures reflect important and persistent health status concerns (1) for which there is not a well-established (i.e., effective) prevention or intervention method, (2) for which no specific improvement is expected within the next five years, and (3) for which sudden changes in prevailing levels or trends would require immediate investigation due to their unexpected nature. Further, good health utilization monitoring measures include those (1) for which the determinants of utilization are not well established, (2) for which no specific improvement in utilization is expected within the next five years, and (3) for which sudden changes in prevailing levels or trends would thereby require immediate investigation. Clearly, the selection of measures of performance should be based on a well-conceived and researched plan that offers a reasonable hope for success. Alternatively, the selection of monitoring measures should reflect an appreciation of current important but unresolved public health problems, tempered by a realistic understanding of current limitations to effect immediate changes.

Examples of poor performance health status measures but good monitoring measures include congenital anomalies and obesity. Little if any change has been observed in the incidence of congenital anomalies during the last two decades and the prevalence of obesity is actually increasing in the United States. Until more effective approaches emerge to address these important risk factors for infant mortality and chronic illness, it is unlikely that states will be able to "perform" positively in these areas.

Indicators for Use in Resource Allocation and Funding Formulas

The focus on performance and accountability leads inevitably to a discussion of funding decisions. The use of funding formulas in the public health field has gathered increasing interest in recent years. Though resources have typically been allocated based on need, resource allocation may become more closely tied to performance in the future. The purpose of employing a funding formula is to provide a rational and more objective basis for equitably distributing funds and allocating resources among geopolitical subdivisions to supplement existing core public health programs and to fill gaps in service.

The basic components of funding formulas are indicators of (1) population health status, (2) health service and system resources, (3) health services utilization, and (4) poverty or socioeconomic status. The inclusion of health status and health utilization indicators provides a strong basis for evaluating the impact of programmatic efforts from one year to the next among the geopolitical areas of a state or geographic region. The direct linkage of the goals and objectives of programs to the funding allocation process is one of the strengths of the use of funding formulas.

The selection of indicators to include in a funding formula entails an intense political process, the results of which could potentially impact jobs and services. The basic principles that guide the selection of indicators for use in funding formulas are similar to those used to select need and performance indicators. Again, these include simplicity, stability, availability (with an emphasis on timeliness), logical, and broad (and equitable) representation. In addition, funding formulas may take into account performance. Some geographic area may have improved their high-risk indicators through successful program performance. These efforts will need to be maintained in order to keep health status at improved levels. Failure to incorporate rewards for high performance penalizes such programs and may result in future decrements of the achieved gains in health status.

There is no single established method for determining which indicators to select for a funding formula. It is likely that several versions will need to be tried in order to observe their effect on funding allocations. To the extent possible, a priori agreements about what in general should be included will reduce some of the need to tinker excessively with versions containing widely different indicators. The same methods used to reach consensus among stakeholders about need priorities can be used. The temptation is to include numerous indicators in order to give recognition to the many interest groups that might be involved. However, this may not be the best strategy. Multiple indicators of the same overall health status problem or need may actually bias a formula by giving extra weight to one problem where no extra weighting was intended. Instead, it is useful to distinguish those indicators that tap different dimensions of public health problems and eliminate repetitive indicators. Some problems may be viewed as having a different level of importance and the indicators of those problems could be given greater weight. As indicators are typically summed and averaged, this approach is only slightly different in the long run from including multiple indicators that essentially measure the same thing.

Basic Premises of Funding Formulas

After the target population has been defined and enumerated, the first basic premise in implementing a funding formula is that without knowledge of health status, each member of the target group should receive equal funding. In other words, in the absence of knowledge of health status or risk, funds should be allocated on a per capita basis. If there is $100,000 and 1000 individuals in the target population, then funds should be distributed to localities on the basis of $100 per individual in the geopolitical subdivision. The second basic premise in creating a funding formula for allocating resources is that given knowledge of health status or risk disparities, higher risk localities should receive additional funds. Next, given knowledge of available local resources, resource-rich localities should get less funds than resource-poor localities. Given knowledge of performance, localities with improved performance (not the best performance but the most improved performance) should be rewarded for their accomplishment. The final premise is that any change in the allocation of funds should be phased in gradually to avoid major disruptions in local services. Abrupt decreases or increases in funds can create service inefficiencies and can have dramatic political repercussions.

Based on these premises, a typical funding formula for use in resource allocation would have several types of indicators, including those of population size, health status need and risk, resource availability, and performance. Population size indicators recognize that localities with larger populations need proportionally more resources. Population-based allocations ensure some level of funding even to low-need localities so as to maintain critical infrastructure. To consider groups with special needs, e.g., newborns, adolescents, persons with disabilities, or immigrants, separate target populations may be used.

Need-based indicators, reflecting health status problems or health risk characteristics, allow for adjustment of population-based funding to provide additional resources to higher-risk populations. Risk ratio scores can be derived for each locality and the population-based allocation adjusted accordingly. Reallocating funds based on health status and risk assumes that additional funding will result in a positive impact on that part of the high-risk population with ameliorable needs. This assumption implies that the additional funds will result in performance, e.g., a change in the indicator in the near future. That, in turn, is contingent on having handy effective solutions that can be implemented.

Indicators of resource availability allow for adjustment of population-based funding in recognition of differences in the availability of local resources. Similar to risk ratios, resource-ratio scores can be derived for each locality and the population-based allocation adjusted accordingly. As local resource availability may be highly correlated with need at the local level, i.e., wealthy counties may have lower needs, the use of resource availability indicators in resource allocation formulas may be seen as partially duplicative. The inclusion of resource availability indicators may largely reflect the desire either to stimulate local investment (the effectiveness of which may be questionable in any given circumstance) or to placate the political outcries of less affluent areas.

Incorporating performance improvement measures into funding formula allows for adjustment of population-based funding in recognition of recent accomplishments in developing and implementing new or expanded capacities or services or in improving health status or health risk. These indicators should reflect actual net improvement, not simply the absolute level or the absence of need. For those localities with the best health status indicators, achieving 10% improvement beyond current levels is likely to be much more difficult than for those localities with much less advantageous health status levels, where a 10% improvement might only bring them close to the average, not the best, localities. Importantly, the reward for net improvement encourages those behind to catch up and is intended to help reduce wide disparities in health status among localities. If rewards were given to those with the best outcomes, the disparities would likely become greater as the resources allocated on the basis of performance would flow to those with the least need. In effect, the rationale for allocating resources on need would be somewhat countermanded. For those localities with similar health outcome levels, the reward allocation based on net improvement highlights accomplishments and hopefully attracts the attention of less successful localities to consider implementing those activities that may have resulted in the improvement.

The example given in Table 5.1 illustrates how funding formulas are used to allocate resources. This example incorporates indicators of population size, health status, population risk characteristics, and performance. For ease of illustration, this example uses three localities or counties, e.g., county A, B, and C. Each of the indicators for each county is standardized to the state average. This is accomplished by dividing each local indicator by the state average to produce risk ratios. The next step is to sum the standardized risk ratios and divide by the number of risk ratios used. If this summary risk ratio is greater than 1, then the locality has a greater risk than the state average.

In the example, the size of the state target population is 10,000 and varies from 2500 in counties A and C to 5000 in county B. The higher rate of the health status indicator selected for the formula is found in county C (10) and the lowest rate is in county A (6). For county B, 25% of its population has the selected high-risk characteristic. The greatest improvement in performance has been reported by county C (15%). As indicated above, standard risk ratios for each indicator are calculated by dividing each local indicator by the state average, e.g., the health status risk ratio for county A is 0.75 (6/8). Summing up the indicator risk ratios for county A results in a total indicator risk ratio of 2.42, which is less than 3 (the total number of indicators used). Dividing the total indicator risk ratio of county A by the number of indicators used (3) provides the summary indicator risk ratio. If this summary indicator risk ratio is greater than 1, then the locality has a greater risk than the state average. In the case of

Figure 5.1. Funding Formula Example Adjusting Population Size by Health Status, Risk and Performance

	A	B	C	State
Population size (#)	2500	5000	2500	10,000
Indicators				
Health status rate	6	8	10	8
% high-risk population	35	25	35	30
% improved performance	5	10	15	10
Indicator risk ratios (IRR)				
Health status	0.75	1.00	1.25	1.00
High-risk	1.17	0.83	1.17	1.00
Performance	0.50	1.00	1.50	1.00
Total IRR	2.42	2.83	3.92	3.00
Summary IRR (total IRR/3)	0.81	0.94	1.31	1.00
$$$ to be allocated	$2500	$5000	$2500	$10,000
Adjusted allocation $$$	$2025	$4700	$3275	$10,000

county A, the summary indicator risk ratio is less than 1, indicating a lower risk than the state average.

Based on our working premises for funding formula, county A in our example would be allocated $2500 of the statewide appropriate of $10,000 on the basis of population size alone. However, as there is knowledge of health status, risk characteristics, and performance, this initial allocation has been adjusted to $2025 by multiplying the initial $2500 allocation by 0.81, the summary indicator risk ratio.

Another approach to funding is to allocate some percentage of funds based on target population size and then to use the remaining percentage of funds to support efforts in higher-risk and lower-resource localities and to reward improved performance. In the example shown in Table 5.2 total funds were allocated on the following proportions: 50% population size, 25% need (health status), 10% local resource availability, and 15% performance. A slightly different amount of funds are allocated to each county by this approach.

Knowledge of economies of scale and scope are needed to ensure that levels of funding are practical. A $10,000 increase may not be useful, if it is insufficient to purchase needed additional personnel. Further, there may well be a base minimum of funding needed to maintain a program. Funding below that level may be of questionable benefit. We are often faced with localities that have a very small or very large percentage of the target population and widely varying degrees of health status risk. In this case, localities with low risk and a small proportion of the target population are given a minimal level

Figure 5.2. Funding Formula Example Emphasizing Population Size over Risk and Performance

	A	B	C	State
Total $$$	2500	5000	2500	10,000
50% $ population size	1250	2500	1,250	5000
25% $ risk	625	1250	625	2,500
Risk adjusted $$$	468.75	1250	781.25	2,500
($ risk × IRR)	(625 × 0.75)	(1250 × 1.0)	(625 × 1.25)	
10% $ resources	250	500	250	1,000
Resource adjusted $$$	187.5	500	312.5	1,000
($ resources × IRR)	(250 × 0.75)	(500 × 1.0)	(250 × 1.25)	
15% $ performance	375	750	375	2,500
Performance adjusted $$$	187.5	750	562.5	2,500
(IRR)	(375 × .5)	(750 × 1.0)	(375 × 1.5)	
Adjusted allocation $$$	2093.75	5000.00	2906.25	10,000

of funding to maintain base services, while other localities compete for additional funding using a funding formula focused on health status risk level.

Other existing approaches to funding may reflect characteristics of a particular state's public health system. Some states have a centralized system where funding to localities largely comes from the state level. Other states use state monies to supplement local funding. Finally, some funding is very categorical to target specific populations that have a very uneven distribution throughout the state. These three circumstances can lead to variations in approaches.

In situations where substantial funding comes from localities, state money is often used to fill gaps in service, to provide technical assistance, and to help prevent future problems from emerging. Typically, there is insufficient funding at the state level to provide all localities with full funding. Further, some localities are "wealthier" than others and have greater resources at their command to initiate their own programs if they desire. In such cases, counties with relatively advantageous health status, low levels of risk, and high resource availability may get no funding. Where resource availability is high and health status concerns exist, technical assistance funding may be offered. For areas with few resources available, funding for primary prevention efforts may be offered, with additional funds made available based on health status levels. A locality's history of performance adds yet another dimension for consideration when setting funding levels and may suggest specific areas to which funds can be targeted. For example, poor performance in improving ongoing adverse health status levels in high risk, low resource communities may indicate the need for targeted funding, coupled with technical assistance and evaluation support.

The last funding formula premise, that any change in allocation be phased in gradually, should not be overlooked. Once a funding formula and resource allocation scheme is adopted, there may need to be an agreement regarding the amount of change allowed. A 50% reduction in funds to a locality is probably unacceptable to all involved and even major increases in funding may not be productive unless spread out. After deciding what the funding formula should be, it may be necessary to limit the possible change in funding to not more than a certain percentage during the first few years of implementation.

Clearly, much progress is being made developing indicators for needs assessments and for performance. These should be linked via the program responses developed to meet needs and measured for success. While they should also be linked by measurement, they are not necessarily interchangeable, e.g., need may be assessed through indicators of newborn mortality and morbidity, while performance may be assessed by appropriateness of delivery site. As much of the interest in performance is driven by desires for accountability and responsible stewardship, the eventual link to resource allocation decisions can be anticipated and should be considered early. Indicators of need, of performance, and of those factors utilized to ensure equitable funding allocations are not necessarily interchangeable.

Discussion Questions

1. What techniques can you use to ensure the needs of disparate population groups or competing health issues are considered in the needs assessment process? How might you apportion and then allocate your limited resources to address these disparate needs assuming that priorities emerge from each differing area (e.g., the elderly versus children, needs for primary and preventive care versus needs for acute and rehabilitative care)?

2. Concerns have been raised regarding whether the self-selection of performance measures by states and localities will result in a lowering of the bar to ensure positive performance results. What approaches can be used to ensure that performance targets are realistic but also sufficiently challenging to be credible and to result in the improvement of the health status condition of interest?

3. Your needs assessment has identified unintended pregnancy among young women 15–24 as an area of primary concern. Plans have been developed to address this problem. Consider possible measures of performance related to this problem, i.e., those measures you believe you can change and are willing to be judged against. Consider possible monitoring measures, i.e., those measures that reflect persistent ongoing health concerns that you are not directly attempting to change but are important nonetheless.

4. Consider the state of Central Dakota, where the health service providers to the population are for-profit corporations. Assuming the state wishes to allocate resources to "local" areas as baseline funding of essential services, in the form of supplemental funding for specific services, or as technical assistance, how does the availability of local resources (in this case, the resources of the health plans) get taken into account and affect your allocation decisions?

5. Consider the state of Old Virginia. What are the limitations of their very centralized approach to needs assessment, priority setting, and the establishment of performance measures, in the allocation of resources to the local level?

6. Given that your state needs assessment efforts might suggest the need for a major reallocation of resources at the local level, how do you plan for a long-term transition (to minimize disruption) given that needs continually change?

6

Determining and
Developing Solutions
The Importance of Goals and Objectives

*The purpose of needs assessment is not to justify the need for current
programs; instead, it is to discover what programs are needed.*

Data Are Not Enough

At this point in the needs assessment process, we have assembled data relevant
to our needs assessment task, we have identified and engaged a group of constituents to guide us through the process, and we have synthesized all the information available to date into a set of indicators or statements of need as well as
indicators or statements of resources and assets. We have further determined
priorities from among the many needs identified and highlighted community
resources or assets that are worthy of further development. We have also considered indicators of performance and various strategies for allocating resources,
should they become available. At this point, the priority needs identified must
now be translated into plans for action. Accepting that each need is real, what
can and should be done to alleviate the need or to enhance the system response
to the need? This is the point at which program planning actually begins, with
the generation of policy and programmatic options for solutions to identified
priority needs.

Some may believe that the gathering of data and the identification of needs
is where needs assessment ends. We disagree, believing instead that the entire
process, from the very beginnings of a desire to do a better job, to the enactment of a plan of action, is part and parcel of the needs assessment process.

91

Further, data gathering may be viewed as the most difficult part of needs assessment efforts and therefore should consume the majority of the resources. We disagree with this sentiment as well; as much energy should be devoted to the careful consideration of solutions as was devoted to the identification of the problem. If effort is not expended to consider and then select the best solution, it is highly unlikely the needs assessment will yield the high expectations associated with it and improvements in health systems or health status will not be forthcoming. Part of the difficulty is people's tendency to look to what they are already doing as the universe of available "solutions" to the needs identified. Indeed, using needs assessments solely to justify current services, programs, and policies may be an unspoken or blatantly obvious agenda, which should be recognized as an understandable, although not recommended, point of view. It is not uncommon to hear agency directors arguing that they need more of ____ (you can fill in the blank) to address the overwhelming health needs in their communities. While it may be true that the agency needs more environmental sanitarians to promote the safety of the food supply, or more economists to predict trends and suggest corrections in health care costs, or more home health aides to allow elderly and disabled citizens to remain in their homes rather than be institutionalized, if these are the only solutions presented, they appear self-serving and likely are shortsighted. Far better to take a broad view and consider any and all possible strategies, however farfetched, before adopting and advocating any one solution. Clearly, your external constituents and partners are as critical in this stage of the needs assessment process as they were early on in helping suggest avenues of inquiry and in establishing priorities.

The identification of true public health needs, deemed important and relevant by both practitioners and the public, is a complex undertaking but does not in and of itself constitute a "needs assessment." Despite what the term implies, the assessment of needs must include the consideration of solutions to address those needs and the development of a clearly articulated and workable plan to resolve or mitigate needs toward improvements in health. One can assemble all the ingredients deemed necessary to bake a cake; but until one follows all the steps in a recipe and actually makes the cake, there isn't much to serve with ice cream.

The recipes we use in public health are action plans and the action plans are grounded in *goals* and *objectives* based on selected *solutions,* or strategies, that when followed, should result in better health for the population or community of interest. Of course, the level of success of any chosen strategy is a direct function of the likelihood that the strategy will be effective in reducing or ameliorating an identified problem area. Sometimes we already know, from scientific research or the successful experiences of others, the most logical course of action: The threat of an outbreak of a vaccine-preventable disease should trigger a massive immunization campaign; repeated injuries associated with a piece of playground equipment should trigger repair or removal of the offending apparatus; an outbreak of a food-borne illness should trigger a recall of the tainted product. In other cases, however, the need is more subtle, the consequences of a need left unaddressed more distal, or there simply are no obvious strategies apparent: e.g., seeming increases in cancer incidence among children in a community with no known connection among them; random acts of violence in schools; the privatization of public hospitals; denuding the environment in the rapid development of housing subdivisions in burgeoning suburban areas. Obviously the more clearly and specifically the problem can be defined, the more precise the solution that can be derived. (See Chapter 5 for further discussion of developing indicators of need and precision of measurement in describing needs.)

Criteria for Determining Feasible Solutions

Several methods for the consideration and selection of policy and program options by which priority needs can be addressed have been developed. These methods for selecting the best possible solutions to identified needs share the common directive to consider, for any solution suggested, its anticipated level of *effectiveness*, its anticipated level of *efficiency*, and its anticipated social and political *acceptability*. Whether you have the *authority* to carry out any specific solution must also be taken into account.

Effectiveness: Is the solution likely to be effective in resolving or reducing the problem? How likely relative to other possible solutions?

Efficiency: What is the cost-benefit of the solution, i.e., at what cost do we achieve success in meeting the need on a population level? Can we afford this solution?

Acceptability: Will the general public find the solution to be acceptable? Will policymakers support the solution given the public's perception of it?

Authority: Finally, is this "solution" within your area of responsibility and within the purview of your program? Or is your primary course of action to inform and advocate with others about this particular problem?

While it is almost intuitive to consider whether or not something will work at a cost you can afford, the issues of authority and acceptability are equally important in deliberating various potential solutions. Some of the most innovative solutions derived may well be outside your programmatic responsibility or your direct sphere of influence; in such a situation, rather than throw your hands up and say "oh, well, not my problem," remember that your efforts served to identify the problem. Given public health's responsibility to *promote those conditions in which people can be healthy*, your strategy can and should be to advocate with the appropriate entities to see that the problem is at least acknowledged if not immediately and fully addressed.

On the question of acceptability, former mayor of Baltimore Kurt Schmoke and recently the current governor of New Mexico, Gary Johnson, among others have advocated for the legalization, or at least the decriminalization, of drugs. When considering the problem of substance abuse in this country, the associated health and criminal risks, and the attendant law enforcement, imprisonment and treatment costs, legalization to some looks like a highly effective and efficient solution to the problem. Politically and socially, such a solution is almost utterly nonviable. Other "solutions" that are nonstarters in our current sociocultural and political climate include euthanasia, involuntary sterilization, elimination of handguns, prohibition of tobacco or alcohol, rationing of health care, or unlimited access to abortion, though it doesn't take much imagination to contemplate the public health problems some of these "solutions" might very effectively and efficiently address. On a less extreme note, consider such solutions as mandatory seat-belt laws, required school-entry immunizations, fluoridated water systems, motorcycle helmet laws, and workplace safety standards; each of these has been and continues to be fraught with controversy even though the effectiveness and efficiency with which each of these has reduced injury and disease are well documented and difficult to dispute.

On the other hand, extremely popular solutions may be neither effective nor efficient. Public concerns over community water supplies, kindled by enticing advertising campaigns, have led to an explosion in the bottled water industry; yet this relatively new industry is not as well regulated as are municipal water systems. You may be buying the same water you would have gotten out of your own tap. The diet industry is also alive and well promising massive weight reductions and physical fitness with this pill, or that menu plan, or this cream, or that concoction of herbs, or, at the extreme, this surgery. Clearly the American public is anxious to lose weight and willing to pay a lot of money to do so; obviously these are popular but not terribly effective or efficient solutions. Good old-fashioned exercise several times a week coupled with a moderate intake of calories from the major food groups over time will result in weight loss, effectively, efficiently, and quite unpopularly.

You can use these factors, *efficiency, effectiveness, acceptability,* and *authority,* informally in your discussions of each solution proposed, or you can derive mathematical calculations or scores for each one allowing for a more quantifiable explanation for your eventual choice. Here are two options:

Option I: Considering and Selecting Solutions
to Identified Public Health Problems

Consider the effectiveness, efficiency, and acceptability of each solution proposed and rate each of them on a scale of 0 to 100%.

Effectiveness
0--|--20--|--40--|--60--|--80--|--100

Efficiency
0--|--20--|--40--|--60--|--80--|--100

Acceptability
0--|--20--|--40--|--60--|--80--|--100

You could then total the three percentages and divide by 3 for a total score for each individual solution proposed. Authority can be determined later.

Option II: Considering and Selecting Solutions
to Identified Public Health Problems

Alternatively, you could consider the effectiveness, efficiency, and acceptability of each solution proposed and assign them a ranking of High, Medium, or Low.

Effectiveness
Low - - | - - Medium - - | - - High

Efficiency
Low - - | - - Medium - - | - - High

Acceptability
Low - - | - - Medium - - | - - High

As previously, you could then generate an overall ranking for the solution, such that a solution that was deemed highly effective, of medium efficiency, and of low acceptability would be rated a "medium" overall. Authority can be determined later.

As previously mentioned, it is easy to fall into the trap of considering only your own current activities as potential solutions. To help guard against this we advocate that you involve external constituencies in these deliberations. Further, we suggest you consider identifying solutions within different categories or types, such as those identified below:

Possible Solutions to Identified Public Health Needs
- Direct services or clinical approaches
- Financing or purchasing of services
- Regulation or quality assurance
- Education of professionals or the public
- Data gathering, monitoring, surveillance
- Systems development

It is always possible that for a top priority need, a highly effective, cost-efficient, and politically acceptable solution does not exist. In such cases, the ranking of needs should be reexamined in light of the efficacy of the available solutions. We will use an example to illustrate this task. Say the priority need identified is an increase in smoking initiation among adolescents aged 15–17. A number of possible options might be considered including school-based education programs, media campaigns, stronger enforcement of laws restricting sales of tobacco to minors, or tax increases on tobacco products (Table 6.1). Let's examine each one against these four criteria.

In this example, we assume we are the public health department and, through our ongoing surveillance, have identified a change in the previous downward trend in youth smoking toward an increase in young people initiating tobacco use. Other data support this observation and our constituency groups not only identified this as a high priority need area but also strongly support

Table 6.1. Possible Solutions to Increased Adolescent Tobacco Use

Possible solution	Effectiveness	Efficiency	Acceptability	Authority
School-based education	Low	Medium	Medium	Health and education
Media campaign	Low	Low	Medium–high	Health
Law enforcement	Medium	High	Medium	Judicial system
Increased tobacco taxes	Medium	High	Low	Commerce

action to reverse this upward trend. Four solutions have been proposed and as we can see, each one varies in its effectiveness in curbing smoking initiation among young people, in its cost, and in its acceptability to the general public and, by extension, lawmakers. We also see that while the public health department and its constituents are very interested in this area, in only two of the four proposed solutions do we have the authority to assume a direct role.

We would like to think that education in the schools, directed at the target population, would be the most direct approach. Research would suggest, however, that these programs are not as effective as once thought. Further, the population represented by this age group, 15–17, may no longer be in school, as many drop out of high school each year. Finally, the growth in alternative and private schools and in the home schooling movement suggests that it will become increasingly more difficult to reach this target population through schools than in previous years when the vast majority of children and youth attended public schools. This particular solution was judged to be of medium efficiency meaning that school-based education programs done well are not inexpensive; yet, on the other hand, many schools have health education programs in place that could perhaps be enhanced with only a modest infusion of resources. We judged the acceptability to be medium; while our constituency recognizes this as a serious problem and we assume that most parents would prefer their children not smoke, there are members of the community that do not believe schools should be used to provide any information beyond the academic and that it is the parents' job to provide counseling and advice to their children on any health-related matter, so that we can expect some resistance to such a solution, however well intended. Finally, this is clearly an area in which the public health agency has expertise and some authority but this particular solution would require a strong collaborative partnership with the education agency and perhaps other community groups as well.

The second proposed solution, a media campaign, was also judged to be of low effectiveness and because of the costs of comprehensive media campaigns, to be of very low efficiency. On the other hand, media campaigns are typically accepted by the general public, particularly when directed at the smoking behavior of young adults and are popular with policymakers because they are clear evidence of action taken in response to an issue of concern to the public. This is also the only one of the solutions squarely within the responsibility and authority of the public health agency, though to be effective, the health agency should partner with other governmental agencies as well as private marketing firms and broadcast media outlets.

The third solution, to strengthen enforcement of laws restricting tobacco sales to minors, is likely to be more effective than either the school-based education program or a media campaign in that strict enforcement should reduce youth access to tobacco products making it more difficult for them to initiate or continue using tobacco. As these laws already exist in most states and law enforcement officers are aware of and capable of handling violations of this type, such an approach should incur little additional costs, certainly not for the health department, and only modestly for the local law enforcement agency. Such an approach, enforcing existing laws, should not provoke extreme negative reactions, except among tobacco companies and retailers who stand to lose profits due to decreased sales and the risk of fines due to illegal sales, but alone is equally unlikely to excite advocates to the extent that a comprehensive approach would. Not only may retail merchants who profit from the sale of tobacco products comply reluctantly, but also they may exert political pressure to reduce the level of enforcement.

The fourth solution, to increase tobacco taxes thereby pricing the products out of the reach of many adolescents, is a popular approach among some political constituencies, but frightens others who fear the emergence of a tobacco "black market." Though there is some research evidence to suggest that price elasticity is important in determining whether or not youth begin or continue to smoke, the results are mixed. Chronic smokers are not susceptible to price increases and some advocates for low-income populations have criticized this approach as one more regressive tax unfairly shouldering the burden on those of lesser means. While such an approach may be effective and is certainly cost-effective, in the current political climate, the general public and policymakers are hostile to any tax increase, even for apparently noble purposes.

As we often find in public health, a multifaceted, coordinated approach is usually preferable to a single, unidimensional effort. In this case, public health officials might well consider a "systems development" approach in which leaders from education, the media, law enforcement, and commerce are brought together with public health advocates, researchers, and program experts to discuss a partnership to reduce the use of tobacco among youth, a goal no one would deny is laudable.

Determining Goals and Objectives

Which brings us to the next step, the explication of a set of goals and objectives that will serve as your blueprint for action. We have identified a need or set of needs and we have considered and narrowed our choice of possible solutions. If we did not have an overarching goal already, we must go back and consider where it is we are trying to go and from that, devise a framework for our future action steps. *Goals* are essential for articulating a vision and communicating your purpose; *objectives* are essential for communicating your strategy, for guiding decision-making, for allocating funds, and for monitoring and evaluation. When writing goals, one should think big and far into the future. One should think "slogan." Goal statements should be something few people can argue with on their surface. Consider these statements:

Healthy mothers, healthy babies
All children should enter school ready to learn
100% access to health care, 0% disparity in health status
Healthy families, healthy communities
Clean air, clean water, safe food

Goals then, in public health, are broad statements of desired health status, or of expected outcomes. Unlike objectives, which we shall discuss in a moment, goals are not stated in measurable terms nor are they fixed in time. They do provide overall programmatic direction, are political in nature, and suggest an ideal state.

Objectives, derived from goals must be much more specific. Objectives form the framework for program planning, implementation, management, and evaluation. Objectives are written statements that tell us what you intend to do, for whom, over what time period, and to what degree. As such, objectives must be composed of an activity or indicator, a target, and a time frame; objectives must be clear, specific, measurable, limited in time, and realistic; objectives should clarify responsibility; and finally, objectives should be clearly relevant to the mission of the organization—the local environmental protection agency is unlikely to have as an objective to provide more intensive prenatal care services, however much they might care about the effect of the environment on pregnancy outcome.

Well-stated, clear objectives are also absolutely essential not only for monitoring the implementation and the progress of your effort but also for evaluating your success. Objectives help you maintain your focus on the needs you have identified and the outcomes you desire and guide not only your immediate short-term planning but also your long-term strategic planning. Clear objectives enable you to refine the overall direction of your effort, clarify your priorities, reflect your chosen strategies, and provide a framework for program management. Simply put, goals describe where you want to go and objectives describe how you intend to get there and the milestones to be passed along the way.

Typically, and to be most useful, a series of objectives will be devised that emanate from the overall goal but that address various levels of the operation necessary to approach achievement of the goal. These different levels of objectives are also important for monitoring and evaluation as you need to know not only what you intended to accomplish but how you intended to accomplish it. If I am interested in improving the childhood immunization rate or reducing hospital days due to injury, I will set a target and I will engage in a series of activities to help me reach my target. In the fortunate event that I am successful in reaching that target, others will ask me how I did it. In the arena of setting objectives, you are likely to find as many schemas as there are authors who have expounded on the subject. We prefer to keep things simple and referring to the above discussion, suggest you begin with *outcome* and *process* objectives. In any case, objectives should be derived from a thorough analysis of the needs being addressed and the precursors to those needs. Your discussion of potential solutions should have included some consideration of the nature of the needs and the factors associated with them; if not, now is a good time to do this. Also, and we'll keep repeating this, objectives must always be measurable and time-specific.

Outcome objectives clarify what it is you intend to achieve. These are the overarching guideposts to your entire effort. The series of national health objectives first promulgated in the early 1980s are largely outcome-based. Some examples from *Healthy People 2010* are as follows. Within the first Goal, which is "increase quality and years of healthy life," we have

- Increase life expectancy to 77.3 years by 2010, from 75.8 years in 1995
- Increase the percentage of persons reporting good, very good or excellent general health to at least 90% by 2010, from 86.2% in 1993–1996

Within another Goal, "improve the health, fitness and quality of life of all Americans through the adoption and maintenance of regular, daily physical activity," we have

- Increase to at least 30% the proportion of people aged 18 and older who engage regularly, preferably daily, in sustained physical activity for at least 30 minutes per day, from 23% in 1995

- Increase to at least 50% the proportion of young people in grades 9 through 12 who participate in daily school physical education, from 25% in 1995

Within the Goal "promote worker health and safety through prevention," we have

- Reduce work-related injuries resulting in medical treatment, lost time from work, or restricted work activity to no more than 5.2 cases per 100 full-time workers, from 7.4 per 100 full time workers in 1996
- Reduce deaths from work-related homicides to no more than 0.5 per 100,000 workers, from 0.7 per 100,000 in 1996

Within the Goal "every pregnancy in the United States should be intended," we have

- Increase to at least 70% the proportion of all pregnancies among women aged 15–44 that are planned, from 49% in 1995
- Reduce pregnancies among females aged 15–17 top no more than 45 per 1000 adolescents, from 76 pregnancies per 1000 females aged 15–17 in 1994

These are all outcome objectives because they set a target, and they are well-written objectives because they define the population, they provide a baseline, and they include a time frame. Notice how clearly each of these is written—we know exactly what it is they are trying to achieve, for whom, compared to what, and by when.

It is also customary to develop what are called *intermediate objectives*, statements that address the precursors or factors contributing to the overall outcome objectives and that provide more specific direction given the approach you have selected. In our earlier teen smoking example, if we have agreed that a media campaign is to be our chosen strategy, then following the outcome objective to reduce the initiation of smoking teens 15–17 years of age by 10% by 2005, we would state one or more intermediate objectives focused on a media campaign. These might include objectives about the target markets to be reached, the amount of air time to be utilized, and the proportion of survey respondents who recall the message.

It must be emphasized that objectives are harder to write than it may appear. Beware of the following traps:

- Failing to specify a target
  - We will reduce infant mortality in 3 years—to what level?
- Failing to specify a time frame
  - We will reduce infant mortality to 6 deaths per 1000 live births—by when?
- Failing to indicate direction
  - The infant mortality rate will change—probably, but up or down?
- Failing to include a baseline
  - We will reduce infant mortality by 10%—compared to what?
- Confusing the issue
  - We will improve prenatal care use and reduce infant mortality—which is it?
- Being overly ambitious
  - We will reduce infant mortality to zero—nice goal, bad objective (not attainable)
- Being overly cautious
  - We will have one fewer infant death—good, but you can do better
- Giving incomplete information
  - We will match the infant mortality rate of China—really? what is it?

Outcome objectives provide overall direction and specify the results you intend to achieve through your programmatic efforts. Outcome objectives help you communicate the problems that have been identified through your needs assessment and the agreed-on level of change desired. They do not explain what you are going to do to achieve these target levels. For that we need *process objectives*. Process objectives guide our activities and help us communicate what measures we will take to achieve the outcome objectives. We will need to know *what* we did so as to explain *how* we did in terms of movement in the outcome indicator of interest. If physical fitness levels actually increase to the target level by 2010, is it because of a media campaign? worksite health promotion programs? reduced insurance premiums for people who exercise? low-cost fitness centers and new parks in urban areas? or would we have exercised more anyway? (Maybe we have finally tired of television.) We will need to measure both how close we came to our target and how fully we implemented each of the steps articulated in our process objectives. It is in this area that it is critical to understand fully the problem being addressed, risk factors, or precursors for the problem, and any other related issues so that we can be sure to address each of these appropriately. If our goal is "healthy children" and our first outcome objective is to "reduce the infant mortality rate to no more than 5.0 deaths per 1,000 live births by 2010, from 7.6 deaths per 1,000 live births in 1995" (from *Healthy People 2010*), then we might begin with some intermediate outcome indicators such as:

- Increase adequate utilization of prenatal care among pregnant women to 95% by 2005 from 78% in 1996
- Reduce smoking among pregnant women to 15% in 2050, from 22% by 2005 in 1996
- Increase folic acid intake of 0.4 mg per day to at least 80% of women aged 15–44 by 2005, from 30% in 1997

and from these, develop process indicators such as:

- Increase insurance coverage for preconception and prenatal services for 90% of women aged 15–44 by 2005, from 65% in 1996
- Increase public prenatal care clinic hours to include evening and weekend hours in 75% of all clinics by 2005, from 50% in 1995
- At the first prenatal visit, screen 100% of women for tobacco use by 2005 (baseline unknown)
- Refer 100% of women who report using tobacco products to smoking cessation classes by 2005 (baseline unknown)
- In conjunction with the March of Dimes and the retail grocers association, develop and launch, by 2002 a comprehensive public education campaign regarding folic acid targeting women at home, at grocery stores, and at their place of employment
- Provide training on folic acid supplementation during pregnancy to 75% of all obstetrical providers by 2001

Once you have agreed on the process you intend to utilize, and have specified this in process objectives, you can then devise the actual plan, complete with action steps, activities, and tasks to be carried out toward achievement of the objectives and progress toward the goal.

Discussion Questions

1. Imagine that the state of Old Virginia Department of Health has no unit with responsibility for Women's Health and that the local assessments identified women's health as a top priority concern across the state. How likely is it that the state health department officials will agree that this is an area of greatest importance? If they perceive that they have no authority for women's health, with whom should they advocate? What other solutions might you consider to this dilemma?

2. Similarly, assume that the State of New Carolina has identified mental health as a top-priority concern but the health department does not currently operate any mental health programs. Staff are now considering the needs identified within their existing resources. What possible solutions might the staff consider in attempting to address this high priority need?

3. For each of the following "need priorities," consider possible solutions within the framework described above. Rate each one according to your assessment of its likely effectiveness, efficiency, and acceptability and derive a "score." You can use the accompanying table to assist you.
   - Increase in homicides among young minority males
   - Increase in hospitalizations for children with asthma
   - Increase in hip fractures among elderly living in their own homes
   - Increase in binge drinking among college-age adults
   - Increase in farm-related injuries resulting in traumatic brain injury

Possible solution	Effectiveness	Efficiency	Acceptability
Direct services or a clinical approach			
Financing or purchasing of services			
Quality assurance or a regulatory approach			
Education			
Data collection, surveillance, monitoring			
Systems development			

4. Develop a goal statement and some possible objectives for each of the three priority areas identified by the health plans in the state of Central Dakota. Remember to include both outcome objectives and process objectives.

5. The state of New Carolina has created an office of assessment and planning to coordinate these functions across the state. Given that the needs assessment/planning cycle also includes an evaluation function, how might you advocate for the creation of an evaluation unit within the state health department? What arguments would you present in support of your proposal?

7

Effecting Program and Policy Solutions

Education plus action equals successful advocacy.

Up to this point, we have been engaged in a variety of tasks to help inform our decision-making about public health problems in our state or community. We have gathered information; we have considered priorities; we have contemplated solutions; we have agreed on goals; and we have formulated objectives. It is almost showtime! But we have one set of steps remaining; we must gain the necessary authority and resources to proceed with our plans. Amazing as it may seem at this point, our well-formulated and amply justified plans may yet fail to be implemented. We may encounter resistance from within our own agency, from our political leaders, from the legislature, or from the public. We may win approval for the plan but fail to be granted the resources necessary to carry it out. Finally, we may be given only narrow authority and few resources with which to proceed in a limited way. Each of these scenarios is possible, despite your best efforts to engage a cross section of the macrocommunity in your entire needs assessment process. Let us consider ways to promote the success of your efforts.

Organizational Context. First we need to examine the structure and behavior of our organization. This text is clearly biased toward state and local health agencies, but these issues are germane to other public institutions, private hospitals or health care organizations, and community groups. In each case there is a leadership structure accountable for the operation of the organization, whether elected or appointed. In the private sector this is usually a board of trustees and in the public sector it is the legislature or a county council. In either case, the leadership body has fiduciary responsibility for the organization as well as an obligation to ensure that the organization acts in accordance with its mission. So, as we discussed in Chapter 6, determining whether or not the activity you propose is even within the authority of the organization is an essential planning step. Assuming it is, it will be up to your leadership body to determine if your priority stacks up against other competing priorities, if it is consistent with the mission and the direction of the organization, and if the costs are assumable within the resource limitations of the organization. You may be given permission to proceed but asked to identify other sources of funding, e.g., federal or foundation grants, revenues from sales of goods or services, or philanthropic gifts. Regardless, it is now time to sell your proposal so as to implement your plans.

State Government

Hearkening back to Civics 101, we know that in our country, government consists of three branches: the executive, the legislative, and the judicial. At the state level, the governor is the chief executive of the state and all of his or her cabinet agencies comprise the executive branch of government. States may have unicameral (one house) or bicameral (two houses) legislatures and will have a schedule (typically annual or biennial) by which they meet and deliberate matters of policy and matters of budget proposed by the executive branch, their own members, or their constituents. Issues can also be decided by the courts in the case of civil or class-action suits regarding particular health needs and possible solutions. The recent spate of tobacco-related lawsuits is one example of how the judicial branch can become engaged in public health debates, the determination of needs, and the granting of authorities and resources to provide redress to those in need. Typically, programmatic proposals are generated within executive branch agencies and deliberated by legislative bodies. If you are carrying out this needs assessment process from within a state government agency as we have described here, you are part of the executive branch and your proposals for new programmatic initiatives will be presented to the legislature in one of three ways:

- As part of the governor's "package" usually in the form of a request from the agency
- As a bill introduced by a member of the legislature either on behalf of the governor, the agency, or a governmental panel or commission

- As a bill introduced by a member of the legislature on behalf of a constituent or group of constituents

Each of these routes to your garnering the necessary authority or resources to implement your program has its benefits and its risks, largely related to the political climate of the state; the nature of the relationship between the governor and the legislature; the public's perception of the trustworthiness of one, the other, or both; and the nature and scope of competing priorities. You will have to think carefully about the implications of utilizing one route over the other. Depending on how your state works, the decision may not be yours; in some states, all agency proposals come through the governor and are assigned to legislators from within the governor's political party. Of course, if the governor chooses not to include your proposal in his or her package, you may be able to work directly with a member of the legislature of your choosing. Make certain this is allowable within your system! If it is not allowable, then in come the external members of your steering committee or other community leaders with whom you have worked. You can casually mention to them that the proposal was not included in the governor's package and therefore will not be prepared as a legislative bill. *They* can then take the proposal to the elected officials from their legislative districts and ask that it be introduced on their behalf. As long as it has been clear all along that you have involved members of the public in your deliberations, this will not come as a surprise (of course, you've heard the dictum "never surprise your boss"). On the other hand, given the breadth of the constituency you have involved directly in these efforts and the extent of the people who have been made aware of your efforts indirectly, it may be hard to stop the momentum created toward resolving the issue.

Legislative Advocacy

Regardless of how the request is presented to the legislature, mobilizing this constituency for political advocacy at this point is very important. Members of any legislative body deal with myriad issues in any given legislative session and are, on balance, more likely than not to be unfamiliar with your particular issue. They are also likely to vote with either their party or the majority if they have not been asked to do otherwise. It is critical that they hear from you and your constituents, both to inform them of the issue and to urge them to vote for the language or resources you need to do the job. We have heard legislators at the state and local level say that three phone calls on an issue constitutes an overwhelming mandate.

Most legislative bodies at the state level work in similar ways: Bills are introduced by members of the legislative body and are heard in one or more committees, depending on the nature of the bill and its ramifications. It is important to have interested parties testify at committee hearings as this is where the deliberative discussions take place. This is also where opposition will appear, some that you may have been expecting and others of which you may have been unaware. The authors of this text have had the experience of appearing before a committee on what they believed was an innocuous bill only to find a rather large and powerful constituency assembled to fight it. Because you cannot always anticipate these things, it is always best to have people in support of your bill available to testify, even if you believe their testimony will not be needed. Once the bill passes out of committee, it is placed on the calendar and heard by the entire body. Testimony from outsiders is not typically taken at the full chamber hearing, but proponents and opponents may still assemble in the galleries or hallways to make their presence and their wishes known to the members.

As you can see, there are many steps along the way at which contact with legislators is important. It is most important to be speaking with, and informing, key members of legislative committees and powerful members of the senate or house about your issue before it is ever heard. You can and should contact them even before a bill is drafted; once the bill has been prepared; before, during, and after committee hearings; and before, during, and after key votes. Letters and phone calls are fine but personal visits are preferred. Whichever media you choose to use, keep your message simple, brief, and clear. Remember to introduce yourself, remain focused, allow time for questions, extend your appreciation for their consideration (regardless of the outcome of the encounter), and write a follow-up thank you letter. Some examples of the types of contacts you may have with legislators follow:

> Step 1: Greetings Senator/Representative X. I am [calling, writing, meeting with you] to discuss the land next to the river. Our community is very much in need of a park where our children can play safely and where we as families and neighborhoods can gather for social and recreational purposes. This land would be perfect for this use. We understand there has been discussion to build a waste disposal site on this land which we

strongly oppose. Not only would such a facility not meet the needs of the community, but it would further reduce the quality of life in our neighborhoods by increasing large truck traffic down our narrow streets, adding pollutants to our air and water, and creating an eyesore. We have worked hard to build a community that is welcoming and friendly to families and a park would do much to enhance the attractiveness of this community and acknowledge our efforts to make it a better place to live. I urge you to consider our request for a park and to reject any proposal to use that land for a garbage site. Thank you.

Step 2: Dear Senator/Representative X. I am [calling, writing, meeting with] you to urge you to support Senate/House Bill 999: Creation of a Park along the River. Our community has long advocated for a park for our children and our families and we need your support to make this a reality. You have always understood the importance of strong communities and safe neighborhoods for families and your support of this bill would surely demonstrate your ongoing commitment. Thank you.

Step 3: Mister/Madam Chair, Members of the Land Use Committee. I am here today to urge you to approve Senate/House Bill 999: Creation of a Park along the River. With me today are the children of PS 117, the local school district, to share with you the pictures they have made and the poems they have written about their dreams for this park that they so desperately need. I have also prepared a report on the proportion of green space to residential, industrial, and commercial space in our neighborhood versus the four surrounding neighborhoods and you can quickly see that we are already far below the norm in terms of having available to us space in which our children can safely play and we as families in this community can gather for socializing and recreation. Though we understand the argument that the waste facility would bring jobs to the community, our unemployment rate is not so high as to cause us to forego this opportunity to make a better life for our children and their children to come. I know you have already heard from the families in this community, many of whom are here today, to urge you to support this bill. On behalf of them, our children, and our community, please vote for Bill 999. Thank you.

Step 4: Thank you notes to the committee members who supported the bill and those who took the time to meet with you. Remember, you still have a floor vote to go!

Step 5: Letters, calls, or visits to the leadership of the house and/or senate and any members who are not already solidly behind you, to urge their support of the bill when it gets to a floor vote. Arrange to have people at the hearing, not to testify, but simply to be present. You can stand outside the hearing room and distribute leaflets if you like.

The whole point of this is to keep your issue alive, to make sure members of the legislature are informed about your issue, to give them opportunities to ask you questions if they are confused, to make an argument that they can support, and to counter the arguments of others when you can. The point is also to let them know that people care about this issue and will vote or not vote for the elected official in this next election, on this issue. In this regard, it is critical that you not be alone in advocating for this particular program or policy solution *but that the community be with you.* Let's talk a bit about community coalition building.

Community Coalition Building

Coalitions are simply groups of individuals or individual organizations that come together around a common purpose and work toward a shared goal. Coalitions may be enduring, assembled around a broad theme, like "healthy mothers, healthy babies," and working successfully on a series of specific issues as they arise, toward the goal of improved maternal and child health. Other coalitions may be temporary, assembled at one moment in time for one purpose and then dissolved, like the citizens coalition to stop construction of a highway interchange in an environmentally fragile area. Coalitions are very important in policy and program advocacy because they are more powerful as a whole than the sum of their individual component parts. Also, often unique to coalitions, is their ability to assemble groups and people who would otherwise have opposing views. The Catholic archdiocese can be persuaded to join with Planned Parenthood to support an increase in funding for a state family planning program if it will mean fewer abortions. Gun advocates and opponents alike can come together to support an automatic weapons ban to prevent random, and deadly, acts of violence, or to support safety locks to protect children. These types of partnerships are impressive to lawmakers and the more broadly representative a coalition can be, the better your chances of succeeding in your legislative aims.

As we have said all along in this text, it is imperative that those most affected by the actions you may take be brought into the needs assessment process as early as possible. In so doing, you have already formed a coalition that can carry you through the process of enacting the solution you have collectively chosen. Though this group has been your "steering committee," depending on how things are going at this point, your group of external constituents may want to formalize their partnership in a coalition that can be identified as associated with the issue under discussion. Being able to identify yourself as being part of a coalition adds weight to the individual contacts people will have with their elected officials. "I'm Robert Johnson and I live in your District. I'm also a part of the Coalition for a Safer Choctaw County." Coalitions can develop a recognizable identity, a logo, or a message that many people can carry to the legislature. There is definitely strength in numbers; there is even greater strength in diversity, so build your coalition thoughtfully.

Advocacy

Advocacy simply means pleading the case of another. In public health advocacy, we are typically speaking on behalf of a community or a group of constituents, around a particular issue or set of related issues. While we generally think of advocacy as being limited to the legislative arena, as already described, advocacy can be targeted at other groups as well and can and should always include an educational component. Advocacy can be directed at public agencies, at private corporations or industry, at employers or schools, or at businesses. People concerned about genetically engineered food targeted not only governments, but also the corporations themselves that were conducting the research and moving products to market. Farmers have been the targets of advocacy efforts to reduce the presence of chemicals in foods as a result of feeding practices or medical treatments of animals, such as antibiotics, steroids, or growth hormone given to cattle to prevent disease and increase milk production. Advocates have put pressure on the pharmaceutical industry to make more affordable the drugs necessary for persons with HIV or AIDS living in developing countries where the resources are simply not available, for example, in sub-Saharan Africa. Advocates have worked to improve the conditions of school facilities in poorer neighborhoods, or to provide more comprehensive services to children with special health needs including those with behavioral and emotional disorders.

You can invite known advocates to participate in your process or you can stimulate the emergence of new advocates based on the results of your needs assessment. Advocates with the energy and the passion to pursue an agenda can be invaluable to you in communicating the needs and the plan; in developing and providing educational materials or programs; in working with the media; in lobbying the legislature; and in supporting your efforts through the implementation and evaluation phases.

Responsible advocacy is based on the best information available, so your needs assessment process will be of benefit to the advocates, just as their activism is of benefit to you. It is also important to monitor the impact of advocacy efforts to determine which are more successful and to make sure that such efforts do not result in unintended consequences. A legislator in Maryland in the early 1980s was persuaded by a group of women's health advocates that prenatal care was essential in the prevention of poor pregnancy outcomes. He was impressed by data linking the lack of early and regular prenatal care to preterm birth and low birth weight and by the resultant costs associated with babies born too early and too small. Unfortunately, he was not presented with an acceptable, efficient, and effective solution, and left to his own devices, he concocted his own. Several days later these same advocates were dismayed to learn that this legislator had introduced a bill fining and jailing women who failed to keep prenatal care appointments! While the *need* had been made clear to him, the *solution* had not. Responsible and thorough advocacy is data-based and addresses all aspects of the issue at hand. It also adheres to some simple but important rules. We close this chapter with the American Public Health Association's Top Ten Tips for Advocacy.

Top Ten Tips for Advocacy

1. Get to know your legislators well
2. Establish a relationship with your elected officials
3. Acquaint yourself with the staff members of legislators and appropriate committees
4. Learn the legislative process and understand it well
5. Identify fellow advocates and partners and seek ways to work together
6. Be open to negotiation
7. Be polite, remembers names, and always thank those who help you
8. Be honest, straightforward, and realistic; never lie to or mislead a legislator
9. Timing is everything for successful participation in the legislative process
10. Be sure to follow-up with legislators and their staff; always send a thank you note

(Adapted from *APHA Advocates Handbook: A Guide for Effective Public Health Advocacy*, American Public Health Association, 1015 15th Street, NW, Washington, DC 20005)

Discussion Questions

1. In none of our case examples does the governor's office interfere with the state health agencies' needs assessment and planning efforts, though in reality, this happens quite frequently. Consider how you would respond to a request from the governor's office to develop a plan and present it to the legislature with a request for funding, on an issue that never emerged in your needs assessment efforts. Now consider the same scenario but with an issue that did emerge but was soundly rejected by your steering committee. Finally, consider this same scenario but with an issue that you have deep personal feelings about and do not believe you could present to the legislature without compromising your personal values.

2. Recalling our discussion in Chapter 4 on communication, what other strategies might the advocates for the park along the river use to bring attention to this issue beyond the legislative action they are taking?

3. Data privacy issues are becoming of increasing concern to the public, particularly given the growth of the Internet and the extraordinary technological ability companies and agencies have to amass large amounts of information on individuals. Your needs for data may well collide with these data privacy concerns. How might you communicate your needs for data and garner public support for the collection of data on individuals in support of public health needs assessments?

4. You have been contacted by a powerful member of the state legislature who is preparing a bill requiring proof of varicella (chicken pox) vaccination for entry to preschool in your state. He has scheduled a hearing in two weeks. In that time period, what data will you assemble for the committee's review? How might you obtain public opinion on this issue to include with your testimony?

8

The Needs Assessment Team

Ideally, needs assessment is an ongoing exercise, valued as much as budget reconciliations and employee performance appraisals, and setting program objectives and implementing program plans. While we would view skeptically any publicly funded program that did not maintain accurate accounts, maintain the highest quality employees or engage in relevant program activities, many agencies do not maintain dedicated staff for "needs assessment" functions. Rather, when it is time to do the needs assessment, existing staff are assigned specific duties, consultants are brought in, or, rarely, an expert is hired, but only temporarily. Given the fiscal realities of public programs it is often hard to justify a full-time employee dedicated to needs assessment activities. How then can you assemble the best possible team to ensure the integrity and quality of your needs assessment efforts?

We have described in these pages a comprehensive approach to needs assessment, one that recognizes and values the roles of many different disciplines and segments of the community in its successful execution. It should be obvious then that no one individual can adequately address the myriad components of a needs assessment and that a team approach is not only more effective but also eminently more practical. Still, one critical member of the needs assessment team is the *leader*. Behind every successful needs assessment effort there is someone who assumes a leadership role: coordinating, collaborating, garnering resources, communicating, and otherwise gently guiding the work of the needs assessment team. We have heard these individuals referred to as the "keeper of the plan," or the "champion," or the "owner of the process." By whatever name, someone must assume the responsibility for the total effort, including the eventual connection between the identification of needs and subsequent action to address them.

A good needs assessment team is a good program management team. Both rely on data for planning, monitoring, and evaluating; solid communication strategies for promoting policy and program initiatives; partnerships with other agency personnel, outside institutions, and communities; advocacy to support overall efforts; and mutual interdependence among all members of the team.

What constitutes a good needs assessment team? We offer the following suggestions for your consideration. Remember, that while it is perhaps ideal to have all of this talent assembled within your organization, you can also look for it outside your unit and capitalize on the opportunity to build or enhance some new partnerships.

Assembling the Needs Assessment Team

- *The Program*. Knowledge of the program area, its statutory basis, its history and philosophy, past trends and future opportunities, is critical to the success of needs assessment efforts. Few programs function well in the absence of staff knowledgeable about the mission, purpose, and functions of the program. The same is true of needs assessment. Placing the identification of needs, the engagement of the community, the search for solutions, and the enactment of a plan in the overall context of program goals is essential for an efficient and successful needs assessment process. This particular knowledge is usually present within existing staff. Other resources include professionals from within the program area who are employed by the federal government at the national or regional level; technical consultants retained expressly to provide guidance in program development; or academicians who study the particular area.
- *The Data*. Clearly, knowledge of databases, data collection methods, data analysis and interpretation, and data display and reporting is essential. In the absence of complementary program knowledge, however, data knowledge alone is insufficient and potentially dangerous. Again, such skill may well exist within your unit, or elsewhere in the health department. It may also exist in a state demographer's offices or within other state agencies. University researchers are skilled in this area and may also have graduate students eager to apply their skills in various aspects of data management. Universities may also have survey research units that include professionals with expertise in survey design, item construction, and data interpretation in addition to the avail-

ability of actual survey administration. Consultants are also available to assist, though are most effective when there is someone on-site with whom they can work directly and who can retain the knowledge provided for future endeavors.

- *Communications.* As noted in Chapter 4, communication specialists are essential to a successful needs assessment process. Persons trained in health education, social marketing, or public relations are often particularly useful in this area. Professionals with these skills may exist in the health agency, or depending on how the state or community is organized, in departments of education or school systems. Alternatively, community-based organizations may employ health educators or other communication specialists to help them get their messages out, or to counsel clients. Again, academicians are available as are consultants.
- *Advocacy and Coalition Building.* As we have stated repeatedly in these chapters, it is absolutely essential to engage the community in every step of your efforts, from initial planning, through the identification of needs and strengths and the determination of priorities, to the enactment of the plan. You may have an expert in community development in your agency or you may have to seek such expertise outside. Many advocacy groups have been formed around public health issues, the most obvious being your state public health association. Most states will have one or more advocacy groups organized around environmental issues, children, health care access, particular ethnic groups, the elderly, the homeless, persons with disabilities or mental illness, or responsible government. Any of these, among others, can be your ally and can provide you not only with direct support but also with knowledge and expertise around community organization and development.
- *Policy Development and Legislative Affairs.* Chances are your agency has a legislative liaison, or someone responsible for governmental affairs or policy. If it comes to the point where your plan requires statutory authority or an allocation of funds, you will need the help of such persons. Again, it would be wise to invite them to work with you early. Depending on how your state or your agency chooses to conduct its business, it may be possible for you to invite either legislators or members of their staff directly to participate in the entire needs assessment process. University faculty in public health, public policy, political science, law, or governmental studies can be particularly helpful in this arena, though your more likely allies are professionals within your own system.

- *The Community.* No needs assessment team is complete, however many professionals of various disciplines it contains, without the active participation of the target population and the community within which all needs assessment activities will be undertaken. This group of team members is absolutely essential throughout the entire process, and includes everyone from civic, business, and religious community leaders, to health care providers, employers, educators, community based organizations, and members of the public at large. The perspectives these team members bring are critical in the identification of needs and the interpretation of data; in the determination of priorities and the deliberation about solutions; and in the implementation of chosen strategies. Ultimately, your success or failure rests on them, regardless of the extent and level of expertise that went into the process, for it is the community that will decide if the promises were kept and the needs addressed. The community keeps you honest and requires that you remain mindful of the ultimate goal: protecting and promoting the public's health.

Putting the Needs Assessment Team to Good Use

Utilizing a needs assessment team effectively requires attention to the process. While this entire volume is devoted to description and discussion of this process, several knowledgeable persons before us have considered the elements of needs assessments that foster success and have summarized them succinctly. One group in particular, Project SERVE, based in the Massachusetts Health Research Institute, Inc., suggested several characteristics of planning and policy development in the development of programs for children with special health care needs, a population of interest to public health professionals because of the complexity of their needs and the inadequacies of our service systems to address those needs (Epstein *et al.*, 1987). They suggest the following, modified slightly for this application:

- *Public–Private Collaboration.* Public health agencies have long recognized the benefits of working in concert with private sector health agencies as well as with sister public agencies. Engaging others is the only rational approach to addressing the myriad factors that inhibit or promote health within communities. Needs assessment, program planning, and policy development is no different and needs to involve others from the outset.

- *Interdisciplinary Steering Committee.* Again, broad representation is highly desirable on the steering committee(s) assembled to guide a needs assessment exercise. Diversity in professional disciplines represented as well as in community organizations and institutions is critical.
- *Active, Participatory Group Process.* Many difficult decisions will be made through the course of a needs assessment effort. It is important to ensure full participation by all of the members of the steering committee. Some of the techniques available to support participatory decision-making include the nominal group process in which committee members each take turns stating their positions, or "voting" on their top priorities; the Delphi approach where several iterations are used to narrow a list to those issues deemed most critical; assigning homework to committee members to address specific issues and then circulating these to other members; assigning subcommittees to work out specific issues within the larger set of issues or perhaps to draft position papers on specific topics; and conducting in-depth interviews with members to elicit their opinions and to seek points of consensus when these do not emerge in open forums or large group discussions.
- *Acknowledged Leadership.* As stated earlier, it is essential that someone be designated or emerge as the acknowledged leader of the process to ensure it continues to move forward. This may be someone with professional stature and recognized skill in the area of needs assessment, or it may be a charismatic leader from among the members who accepts this responsibility. Regardless, leadership is essential to the successful conduct and completion of the needs assessment process.
- *Consumer Participation.* When relevant, the direct input of service clients or purchasers is critical; when the issues are not germane to individual clients but to the population at large, then community participation is essential.
- *Commitment to Organizational and Policy Changes.* Needs assessments imply a promise of change: If you cannot keep the promise, do not do the assessment. It is reasonable to establish a tentative implementation time-line at the beginning of the needs assessment process, both to make explicit your willingness to enact program or policy changes found necessary through this process, and to provide you the time to do so successfully.

- *Confidence in Local Availability of Information and Talent.* While many are persuaded of the need for outside professional expertise, or feel that the information they need is only credible if it comes from an official source, successful needs assessment teams know that the best information and expertise they have is right in their own communities and they optimize it whenever possible. Locally derived information and talent can and should be supplemented with other documentation and professional consultation, but never substituted.
- *Encouragement of the Ideal.* While practicality dictates a prudent approach to program planning and policy development, needs assessments flourish when people are stimulated to think creatively. The ideas generated will inform a better process in the long run and may suggest areas for long-term planning or future needs assessment efforts.

The Importance of People

A recent study by the Public Health Foundation (Laura Giordano, personal communication, 1998) designed to examine factors that enhanced or hindered data sharing across different governmental agencies concluded that the most important factor in successful interagency data sharing efforts was whether or not the people responsible for data within each agency had an established relationship. Other potential barriers, from incompatible hardware and software, to conflicting confidentiality policies could all be worked out if the people involved liked and trusted each other and worked well together. Never underestimate the power of people who work with you and support you or those whom you do not invite to participate and who work actively against you. Engaging likely constituents, whether they are for or against you, as early in the process as possible, is absolutely essential to the success of the entire needs assessment effort. Though it requires a seemingly extraordinary investment of time and energy, the payoffs are enormous. And, of course, the costs of not engaging your partners early can be more than you can afford to pay.

Discussion Questions

1. Considering the cases of the states of New Carolina and Central Dakota, both of which involved the recruiting of new staff to support the needs

assessment and planning efforts being discussed, who do you believe is missing from these teams? Do you believe it was necessary to hire these individuals or might this expertise have been garnered somewhere else? How difficult or easy do you believe it is to hire people with these particular talents?

2. Given that the state of Old Virginia appears to be entirely relying on existing staff, given your knowledge of state health agencies, in what areas do you believe they may be weak? Where might they find the expertise you feel they might lack? How might they engage these experts to work in partnership on this needs assessment plan?

3. To what extent does organizational structure, culture, and historical practice influence group participation, interaction, and success in the conduct of needs assessments that entail consideration of multiple programs and diverse populations? What strategies might you utilize to overcome some of these institutional barriers to collaboration and cooperation?

9

A Call for Leadership

Having now completed your review of this textbook and having considered the many issues involved in comprehensive needs assessments, you may find yourself encouraged and motivated or you may find yourself daunted by the prospect of such an enormous task. While these efforts may seem challenging beyond your capabilities, be assured that this can be done and it can be done well. We also hope you leave this review with an understanding that not only can this be done, it must be done.

Without ongoing, sustained effort at assessing and documenting needs and performance, agencies are left doing what they have always been doing, probably very comfortably, but with no knowledge of whether what they have been doing is appropriate or necessary. Discussions of new initiatives are based on the opinions of staff, or the demands of external constituents, neither of which are grounded in substance or fact. If you are not questioning what you are doing, if you are not actively seeking information from others, you are not being challenged to create and test new ideas. When faced with either an unexpected increase or decrease in your resources, you will not know which new direction to explore or which activity to end. You will become caught in personalities, in politics, and in public opinion and be left in an indefensible position. Needs assessments done and done well not only show you the way, they protect you from the vagaries of a fickle public and a highly politicized government system.

In our experience, the critical factor is *leadership*. But make no mistake, leadership is not reserved for the name at the top of the organizational chart. Leadership can and must be cultivated throughout your organization. Needs assessments in the context presented here, that of an ongoing planning cycle, are complex, high energy tasks, requiring the participation of many individuals working in concert toward a mutual goal of improving the public's health.

To sustain the level of productivity necessary over time, requires an environment that supports innovation and collaboration, and where the leadership of the organization recognizes and rewards this effort. While individual incentives are always welcome, the true test of whether needs assessment efforts are recognized and rewarded is in *how the agency uses them to support change and strive for improvement.*

We consider the following attributes important to the development of leadership within an organization, again noting that leadership can and should rest throughout the team, not only within certain individuals.

- Energy
- Purpose and direction
- Ability to communicate clearly and articulate the mission of the organization
- Enthusiasm and affection
- Excitement
- Strategic thinking
- Risk-taking and courage
- Integrity
- Adaptability and flexibility

While we believe leadership is necessary, it is not sufficient for successful needs assessment efforts. In this book we have highlighted several factors important to meaningful needs assessment efforts. To reiterate a few here, first, needs assessment must be viewed as a shared task built on partnerships between the public health system and the public. Involving the public early and often is critical to gaining the depth of knowledge desired about the community as well as to earning support for the initiatives suggested by the needs assessment. Second, and related to the first, public health exists within a political environment, and needs assessment is the vehicle by which the science is melded with the politics. This is why it is critical to continually reassess the priorities suggested by the data in light of the realities of acceptability of possible solutions to the problems identified by the data. One should never suggest a solution for a problem that has not been clearly described and supported by data. On the other hand, one should never use data alone to bulldoze a solution to a hostile public. Third, as change is inevitable, needs assessments should never be used simply to justify continuing what you are already doing, but rather to suggest to you reasonable modifications to your operations that will allow you to stay in the forefront of public health promotion in your community. Finally, needs assessment demands patience. The process is arduous and it can become tedious, but in the end, you will find the results are worth the wait.

Two stories to illustrate this last point are the following.

The governor of a state was interested in establishing a center for women's health based on some experiences within his family. He "knew" what the focus should be, based on these limited experiences, and asked the commissioner of health to present this proposal to the legislature. The commissioner, exhibiting many of the leadership qualities noted earlier, wandered the corridors of the health department and asked different public health professionals what they believed a center on women's health should be about. Receiving widely conflicting responses, none of which matched the ideas of the governor, she asked for some information on what was known about the status of women's health in the state, and learned that very little could be described from existing databases, beyond pregnancy related conditions and mortality.

Recognizing that a women's health center without a clear mission would not go over well with the legislature and could easily become the subject of ridicule in the public, the commissioner convened a group and charged them with quickly obtaining information from women and from leading experts across the state on the current status of women's health. Facing limited time, staff decided to organize a series of focus groups across the state; to interview key informants, known experts in the field of women's issues (not exclusive to health); to review and summarize the literature; to compile whatever data were available; and to convene a symposium at which participants would be asked to discuss the findings of these data gathering exercises and recommend a mission and priorities for a center on women's health.

To the surprise of many in the health department, who because of history and organizational structure tended to focus on women's health in terms of infectious disease control, family planning and pregnancy, and chronic disease prevention, the overwhelming conclusion of this needs assessment effort was that the primary concerns of women and the associated needs for services in the state were in the areas of mental health and dental health. This information led to the development of a proposal to create a women's health center that would engage in research; design databases to capture information; provide education, technical assistance, and referral; and advance the state of knowledge in these topical areas. The results of this needs assessment were clearly worth the effort required to obtain them.

In another state, the governor was informed that several million dollars unspent from two federal health-related block grants was available for new initiatives. Knowing that it was nearly time for his state-of-the-state address for the year, he determined that it would be nice to have staff in the health department prepare an initiative around children's health in a particularly high-risk community for him to announce in this address. Staff were instructed to speak to no one about this as he wanted this exciting news to come from him.

Staff diligently pored through all the available databases looking for indicators of health status and health risk that would suggest an appropriate target community, and they found one. Given the myriad problems in this particular community, staff devised a series of programmatic initiatives designed to benefit children and families in this community. Recognizing that health is more than simply the absence of disease, staff took a holistic approach and included interventions targeted at schools, jobs, and recreation in addition to health services and health promotion activities.

Staff also planned a community forum to follow the governor's speech. Key leaders in the community, agency representatives, and the general public were invited to learn more about the proposed initiatives and offer any input they wished into the structure of the overall effort. Staff were pleased with the large turnout at the meeting and approached the podium confidently to present the Child Health Promotion Initiative. Almost immediately, voices in the audience interrupted the presentation. "What are you going to do about the rats?" one participant after another asked. These people had turned out for this meeting because it was the first time in anyone's memory that any representative of the health department had visited the community and they had been trying for years to get someone to attend to their growing problem of rat infestation. Bottom line, they were completely uninterested in anything being suggested until someone attended to what they knew was their most fundamental problem—rodents. This was a case where a little time spent with the community would have avoided the several years of frustration that followed.

Each of these scenarios suffers from one of the fundamental mistakes of needs assessment: only doing it once. Needs assessment is not a task, it is a way of doing business in public health, day after day after day. Think of a seismograph, monitoring activity in the earth's crust for signs of impending earthquakes. Needs assessments done well, done in a continuous way as part of an ongoing planning cycle, serve as the finger on the pulse of the community and allow us to know where our energies are best spent in serving the public's desire to enjoy a state of good health. Leadership to sustain these activities is important and to use the information effectively is essential.

We wish you all the best in your needs assessment activities and know that you can and will be successful. The public is depending on you.

References

Alexander, G. R., Tompkins, M. E., Allen, M. C., and Hulsey, T. C. (1999). Trends in racial differences in birth weight and related survival. *Maternal and Child Health Journal 3*(2), 71–79.

Centers for Disease Control. (1990). Case definitions for infectious conditions under public health surveillance. *Morbidity and Mortality Weekly Report, 39*(RR13).

Centers for Disease Control. (1999). Abortion surveillance - United States, 1996. *Morbidity and Mortality Weekly Report, 48*(SS-4), 1–42.

Centers for Disease Control. (2000). Case definitions for infectious conditions under public health surveillance. Atlanta, GA: Centers for Disease Control and Prevention, Epidemiology Program Office, Report, July 25, 2000.

Connolly, W. B., and Marshall, A. B. (1991). Drug addiction, pregnancy and childibrth: legal issues for the medical and social services community. *Clinical Perinatology 18*(1), 147–186.

Epstein, S. G., Taylor, A. B., and Halberg, A. S. (1987). *New directions: A needs assessment and state planning model for children with special health care needs.* Boston: Project SERVE.

Family Health Outcomes Project. (1997). *Selecting health indicators for public health surveillance in a changing care environment.* University of California at San Francisco.

Feldman, P., Gold, M., and Chu, K. (1994). Enhancing information for state health policy. *Health Affairs*, 237–250.

Health Resources and Services Administration. (1999). *Maternal and child health services block grant application guidance.* Rockville, MD: U.S. Department of Health and Human Services.

Henshaw, S. K., and Forrest, J. D. (n.d.). *Women at risk of unintended pregnancy, 1990 estimates: The need for family planning services, each state and county.* New York: Alan Guttmacher Institute, 6–10.

Hulsey, T. (1986). *Funding formulas for maternal health, child health, teenage pregnancy, and family planning programs in Maryland.* Baltimore, MD: Office of Planning and Analysis for Health.

Institute of Medicine. (1988). *The future of public health.* Washington, DC: National Academy Press.

Kettner, P. M., Moroney, R. M., and Martin, L. L. (1990). *Designing and managing programs: An effectiveness-based approach.* Newbury Park, CA: Sage Publications.

Klerman, L. V., Rosenbach, M., and Jones, K. (1984). *Need indicators in maternal and child health planning.* Unpublished manual, Florence Heller Graduate School for Advanced Studies in Social Welfare, Brandeis University, Waltham, MA.

Krueger, R. A. (1994). *Focus groups: A practical guide for applied research.* Newbury Park, CA: Sage Publications.

Maslow, A. (1954). *Motivation and personality.* New York: Harper & Row.

Maternal and Child Health Model Working Group. (1997). *MCH model indicators: Final report.* Washington, DC: Maternal and Child Health Bureau, Health Resources and Services Administration.

McKillip, J. (1987). *Need analysis: Tools for the human services and education.* Applied Social Research Methods Series, Vol. 10. Newbury Park, CA: Sage Publications.

Moseley, R., and Bell, C. (1991) Prenatal screening for illegal drugs: Dilemma for the nurse-midwife. *Journal of Nurse Midwifery, 36*(4), 245–248.

National Center for Health Statistics, Division of Vital Statistics. (2000). *Report of the panel to evaluate the US standard certificates and reports.* Hyattsville, MD: National Center for Health Statistics.

National Committee for Quality Assurance. (1996). *Health plan employer data and information set (HEDIS 2.5).* Annapolis Junction, MD: Author.

Newacheck, P. W. (1991). *State estimates of the prevalence of chronic conditions among children and youth.* San Francisco: Institute for Health Policy Studies.

Newacheck, P. W., and Taylor, W. R. (1992). Childhood chronic illness: Prevalence, severity, and impact. *American Journal of Public Health, 82*(3), 364–371.

Peoples-Sheps, M., Guild, P. A., Farel, A. M., Cassady, C. E., Kennelly J., Potrzebowski, P. W., and Waller, C. J. (1998). Model indicators for MCH: An overview of process, product and applications. *Maternal and Child Health Journal, 2*(4), 241–256.

Pickin, C., and St. Leger, S. (1993). *Assessing health need using the life cycle framework.* Buckingham, England: Open University Press.

Roth, J. (1990). Needs and the needs assessment process. *Evaluation Practice, 11*(2), 141–143.

Taylor, H. (1997). *Public health: Two words few people understand even though almost everyone thinks public health functions are very important.* New York: Louis Harris and Associates.

United States Congress. (1935). Grants to states for maternal and child welfare. *Social Security Act,* Public Law 271, 74th Congress. 49 US Statutes, 633, Title V.

United States Congress. (1981). Preventive health and health services block grants to states. *Public Health Service Act, as amended, Omnibus Budget Reconciliation Act of 1981,* Public Law 97–35, Title XIX, Section 1905.

United States Congress. (1993). *Government Performance and Results Act,* 103rd Congress, Public Law 103–62.

United States Congress. (1996). *Health Insurance Portability and Accountability Act,* 104th Congress, Public Law 104–191.

United States Department of Health and Human Services. (1982). *Report to the Congress on the study of equitable formulas for the allocation of block grant funds for preventive health and health services, alcohol and drug abuse and mental health services, maternal and child health services.* Washington, DC: U.S. Government Printing Office.

United States Department of Health and Human Services (1989). *Reducing the health consequences of smoking—25 years of progress: A report of the surgeon general.* Washington, DC: U.S. Government Printing Office.

Further Reading

Aberndroth, T. W. (1993). End-user participation in the needs assessment for a clinical information system. *Annual Symposium on Computer Applications in Medical Care, 15,* 233–237.

Altschuld, J. W. (1993). The utilization of needs assessment results. *Evaluation and Program
Planning, 16*(4), 279–285.

Association for the Care of Children's Health. (1993). Advocacy . . . professing one's convic-
tion. *The ACCH Advocate, 1*(1), 4–-12.

Bardsley, M., Jenkins, L., and Jackson, B. (1998). For debate: Local health and lifestyle surveys—do the results justify the costs? *Journal of Public Health Medicine, 20*(1), 52–57.

Bauer, E. I., and Harger, P. S. (1994). Assessing community needs. *Health Progress, 75*(1), 54–
59.

Bell, R. A., Sundel, M., Aponte, J. F., Murrell, S. A., and Lin, E. (1983). *Assessing health and
human service needs: Concepts, methods and applications.* Community Psychology Series
Vol. VIII. New York: Human Sciences Press.

Bennett, E. J. (1993). Health needs assessment of a rural county: Impact evaluation of student
project. *Community Health, 16*(1), 28–35.

Bennington, A. C., and Davies, B. (1980). Territorial need indicators: A new approach (part I).
Journal of Social Policy, 9(2), 145–168.

Bloom, B. S., and Fendrick, A. M. (1987). Waiting for care: Queuing and resource allocation.
Medical Care, 25(2), 131–139.

Blum, R. W., Resnick, M. D., Harris, L., and Bennet, S. (n.d.). *Conducting an adolescent health
community needs assessment.* Minneapolis, MN: National Adolescent Health Resources
Center.

Bosanac, E. M., Petersen, V. J., Forren, G. L., and Baranowski, T. (1982). A resource inventory
approach to needs assessment. Examples from a statewide hypertension control program.
Social Science and Medicine, 16, 1301–1307.

Bosworth, T. W. (1999). *Community health needs assessment: The healthcare professionals' guide
to evaluating the needs in your defined market.* New York: McGraw–Hill.

Bowman, C. (1992). Community and medical staff collaborate in needs assessment. *Health
Progress, 73*(8), 72–75.

Boyd, L. N. (1992). The needs assessment—Who needs it? *Roeper Review, 15*(2), 64–66.

Brazil, K. (1993). Mental health needs of children and youth with learning disabilities: Overview of a community needs assessment. *Evaluation and Program Planning, 16*(3), 193–
198.

Brindis, C. D. (1991). *Adolescent pregnancy prevention: A guidebook for communities.* Palo
Alto, CA: Stanford Health Promotion Resource Center.

Bruner, C., Bell, K., Brindis, C., Change, H., and Scarbrough, W. (1994). *Charting a course: Assessing a community's strengths and needs*. New York: National Center for Service Integration.

Callahan, D. (1990). Needs, endless needs. *What kind of life? The limits of medical progress* (pp. 31–68). New York: Simon & Schuster.

Centers for Disease Control. (1992). Rapid health needs assessment following Hurricane Andrew, Florida and Louisiana 1992. *Morbidity and Mortality Weekly Report, 41*(37), 685–688.

Centers for Disease Control. (1993). Comprehensive assessment of health needs 2 months after Hurricane Andrew, Dade County Florida 1992. *Morbidity and Mortality Weekly Report, 42*(22), 434–437.

Child and Adolescent Health Policy Center, The Johns Hopkins University, School of Hygiene and Public Health, Department of Maternal and Child Health. (1995). *Child health systems primary care assessment: Community self-assessment guide*. Baltimore.

Committee on Health Care for Homeless People, Institute of Medicine. (1988). *Homelessness, health, and human Needs*. Washington, DC: National Academy Press.

Dean, K. (1993). *Population health research*. Newbury Park, CA: Sage Publications.

Delgado, J. L., and Estrada, L. (1993). Improving data collection strategies. *Public Health Reports, 108*(95), 540–545.

DeVillaer, M. (1990). Client-centered community needs assessment. *Evaluation and Program Planning, 13*, 211–219.

Donaldson, C. (1993). Needs assessment: Developing an economic approach. *Health Policy, 25*(1/2), 95–108.

Eng, E., and Blanchard, L. (1991). Action-oriented community diagnosis: A health education tool. *International Quarterly of Community Health Education, 11*, 93–110.

Farel, A. M. (1994). Needs assessments in MCH programs. In H. M. Wallace, R. P. Nelson, and P. J. Sweeney (Eds.), *Maternal and child practices* (4th ed., pp. 141–148). Oakland, CA: Third Party Publishing.

Farel, A. M., Margolis, L. H., and Lofy, L. J. (1994). The relationship between needs assessments and state strategies for meeting Healthy People 2000 objectives: Lessons from the maternal and child health services block grant. *Journal of Public Health Policy, summer*, 173–185.

Gable, C. B. (1990). A compendium of public health data sources. *American Journal of Epidemiology, 131*, 381–394.

Gortmaker, S. L., and Sappenfield, W. (1984). Chronic childhood disorders: Prevalence and impact. *Pediatric Clinics of North America, 31*(1), 3–18.

Governor's Planning Council on Developmental Disabilities. (1992). *Minnesotans speak-out!* St. Paul: Governor's Planning Council on Developmental Disabilities.

Guyer, B., Schor, L., Messenger, K. P., Prenney, B., and Evans, F. (1984). Needs assessment under the Maternal and Child Health Services Block Grant: Massachusetts. *American Journal of Public Health, 74*(9), 1014–1019.

Harlow, K. S., and Turner, M. J. (1993). State units and convergence models: Needs assessment revisited. *The Gerontologist, 33*, 190–199.

Havens, H. S. (1981). Program evaluation and program management. *Public Management Forum*, 480–485.

Helms, W. D., and Isaac, M. (1991). *Review of needs assessment approaches*. Washington, DC: Alpha Center.

Herman, J. L., Morris, L. L., and Fitz-Gibbon, C. T. (1987) *Evaluator's handbook*. Newbury Park, CA: Sage Publications.

Holt, K.A. (Ed.). (1991). *Needs assessment and beyond: 1991 state adolescent health coordinators conference proceedings.* Washington, DC: National Center for Education in Maternal and Child Health.

Huettner, J. (1992). *Small area health needs assessment at the community sub-census tract level, an alternative to CDC's PATCH.* Presentation at APHA, Washington, DC.

Iutcovich, J. (1993). Assessing the needs of rural elderly. *Evaluation and Program Planning, 16,* 95–107.

Johnson, D. E., Meiller, L. R., Miller, C. L., and Summers, G. F.(Eds.). (1987). *Needs assessment: Theory and methods.* Ames: Iowa State University Press.

Johnson, K., Hughes, D., and Rosenbaum, S. (1988). Advocacy for women and children. In H. M. Wallace, G. Ryan, and A. C. Oglesby (Eds.), *Maternal and child health practices* (3rd ed., pp. 203–213)),. Oakland, CA: Third Party Publishing.

Joint Commission of Accreditation of Healthcare Organizations. (1990). *Primer on indicator development and application: Measuring quality in health care.* Oakbrook Terrace, IL: Author.

Joint Commission on Accreditation of Healthcare Organizations. (1992). *Development and application of indicators for continuous improvement in perinatal care.* Oakbrook Terrace, IL: Author.

Kaufman, A., and Waterman, R. (1993). *Health of the public, a challenge to academic health centers: Strategies for reorienting academic health centers.* San Francisco: Health of the Public Program.

Kehrer, B. H. (1993) Seven reasons to evaluate. *Foundation News,* pp. 30-34.

Kennedy, P. (1993). Goal planning, needs assessment and advocacy. *Health Services Management, 89*(3),17–19.

Klerman, L. V., Russell, A. Y., and Valadian, I. (n.d.). *Promoting the health of women and children through planning.* Washington, DC: US Department of Health and Human Services.

Koo, D., and Wetterhall, S. F. (1996). History and current status of the national notifiable diseases surveillance system. *Journal of Public Health Management Practice, 2*(4), 4–10.

Krieger, N., Chen, J. T., and Ebel, G. (1997). Can we monitor socioeconomic inequalities in health? A survey of health departments' data collection and reporting practices. *Public Health Reports; 112,* 481–491.

Lareau, L. (1983). Needs assessment of the elderly: Conclusions and methodological approaches. *The Gerontologist, 23*(5), 518–526.

Lareau, L. S., and Heumann, L. F. (1982). The inadequacy of needs assessment of the elderly. *The Gerontologist, 22*(3), 324–330.

Lauffer, A. (1982). *Assessment tools: For practitioners, managers, and trainers.* Newbury Park, CA: Sage Publications.

Levin, H. M. (1983). *Cost-effectiveness.* Newbury Park, CA: Sage Publications.

Ley, K. (1992). Local needs assessment for workplace literacy programs. *Adult Learning,* pp. 15–16.

Minnesota Institute of Public Health. (1991). *Plan for promoting and supporting breast-feeding in the Minnesota WIC program.* St. Paul: Minnesota Institute of Public Health.

Minnesota Women's Health Initiative. (1994). *Women's Health Initiative.* St. Paul: Minnesota Department of Health.

Misskey, E. (1985). A comparison of three needs assessment methods. *Journal of Nutrition Education, 17*(4), 143–146.

Mohr, L. B. (1992). *Impact analysis for program evaluation.* Newbury Park, CA: Sage Publications.

Monahan, C., and Craik, D. (n.d.). *FOCUS for children: A community planning model to de-*

velop comprehensive, community-based, family-centered care for children with special health care needs (Draft). Chicago: University of Illinois.

Moore, C. M. (1987). *Group techniques for idea building.* Newbury Park, CA: Sage Publications.

Moseley, J. (1993). Needs assessment and rationing in health and social care. *Research Report-Policy Studies Institute, 757,* 18–33.

Moskowitz, J., Stullich, S., and Deng, B. (1993). *Targeting, formula, and resource allocation issues: Focusing federal funds where the needs are greatest.* Supplemental volume to the National Assessment of the Chapter 1 Program. Washington, DC: U.S. Department of Education.

Mulvihill, B., Pass, M. A., Miller, T. M., Mulvihill, F. X., and Klerman, L. V. (1996). Collaborative needs assessment and systems development in Alabama: Process and products. *American Journal of Preventive Medicine, supplement, 12*(4), 14–19.

Nelson, F., Leitheiser, A. T., Hillmer, T., White, K., and Moen, M. E. (1993). The Minnesota HIV services planning project: An assessment of current and future needs for persons living with HIV infection in a low-incidence state. *AIDS & Public Policy Journal, 8*(1), 27–35.

Neuber, K. A. (1980). *Needs assessment: A model for community planning.* Sage Human Service Guides, Vol. 14. Newbury Park, CA: Sage Publications.

North Dakota Department of Human Services. (1991). *North Dakota MCH/crippled children's services combined needs assessment components A, B, and C.* Bismarck: North Dakota Department of Human Services.

Payne, S. M. C., and Strobino, D. M. (1984). Two methods for estimating the target population for public maternity services programs. *American Journal of Public Health, 74,* 164–166.

Peoples-Sheps, M. D., and Miller, C. A. (1983). Monitoring and assessment in maternal and child health: Recommendations for action at the state level. *Journal of Health Politics, Policy, and Law, 8,* 251–276.

Peoples-Sheps, M. D., Siegel, E., Guild, P. A., and Cohen, S. R. (1986). The management and use of data on maternal and child health and crippled children: A survey. *Public Health Reports, 101*(3), 320–329.

Peoples-Sheps, M. D., Byars, E., Rogers, M. M., and Finerty, E. J. (1990). *Using objectives for program planning.* Available from the School of Public Health, University of North Carolina at Chapel Hill.

Peoples-Sheps, M. D., Rogers, M. M., and Finerty, E. J. (1990). *Monitoring progress towards achievement of objectives.* Available from the School of Public Health, University of North Carolina at Chapel Hill.

Peoples-Sheps, M. D., Farel, A., and Ahlowglia, I. (1994). *Companion document to the five-year MCH application guidance.* Rockville, MD.

Peoples-Sheps, M. D., Guild, P. A., Farel, A. M., Cassady, C. E., Kennelly J., Potrzebowski, P. W., and Waller, C. J. (1998). Model indicators for MCH: An overview of process, product and applications. *Maternal and Child Health Journal, 2*(4), 241–256.

Pestano-Binghay, E. (1993). Nutrition education issues for minority parents: A needs assessment. *Journal of Nutrition Education, 25*(3), 144–146.

Poland, M. L., Giblin, P. T., Waller, J. B., and Bayer, I. S. (1991). Development of a paraprofessional home visiting program for low-income mothers and infants. *American Journal of Preventive Medicine, 7,* 204–207.

Pollock, A. M., and Rice, D. P. (1997). Monitoring health care in the United States. *Public Health Reports, 112,* 108–113.

Poole, D.L., and Carlton, T. O. (1986). A model for analyzing utilization of maternal and child health services. *Health and Social Work, summer,* 209–221.

Prescott, N., and De Ferranti, D. (1985). The analysis and assessment of health programs. *Social Science and Medicine, 20*(12), 1235–1240.

Reviere, S. B., Carter, C. C., and Ferguson, C. G.(Eds.). (1996). *Needs assessment: A creative and practical guide for social scientists.* Washington, DC: Taylor & Francis.

Rhodes, J. E., and Jason, L. A. (1981). Community needs assessment. In H. E. Schroeder (Ed.), *New directions in health psychology assessment* (pp. 159–173). New York: Hemisphere Publishing.

Robinson, J., and Elkan, R.(1996). *Health needs assessment: Theory and practice.* New York: Churchill Livingstone.

Roush, S., Birkhead, G., Koo, D., Cobb, A., and Fleming, D. (1999). Mandatory reporting of diseases and conditions by health care professionals and laboratories. *Journal of the American Medical Association, 282*(2), 164–170.

Royce, D., and Drude, K. (1982). Mental health needs assessment: Beware of false promises. *Community Health Journal, 18*, 97–105.

Satin, M. S., and Monetti, C. H. (1985). Census tract predictors of physical, psychological, and social functioning needs assessment. *Health Services Research, 20*, 341-358.

Sciarillo W. G. (1988). Children with specialized health needs in the special education setting: A statewide technical assistance approach. *Infants and Young Children*, pp. 74–84.

Scriven, M. (1990). Special feature: Needs assessment. *Evaluation Practice, 11*(2), 135–144.

Shadish, W. R., Cook, T. D., and Leviton, L. C. (1991). *Foundations of program evaluation.* Newbury Park, CA: Sage Publications.

Smeloff, E. A. (1981). A geographic framework for coordination of needs assessment for primary medical care in California. *Public Health Reports, 96*(4), 310–314.

Steinwachs, D. M. (1989). Application of health status assessment measures in policy research. *Medical Care, 27*, S12–S26.

Stewart, R. (1979). The nature of needs assessment in community mental health. *Community Mental Health Journal, 15*(4), 287–295.

Sullivan, C. (1992). After the crisis: A needs assessment of women leaving a domestic violence shelter. *Violence and Victims, 7*(3), 267–275.

Surles, K. B., and Blue, K. P. (1993). Assessing the public's health: Community diagnosis in North Carolina. *Public Health Reports, 108*, 198–203.

Thacker, S. B., and Stroup, D.F. (1994). Future directions for comprehensive public surveillance and health information systems in the United States. *American Journal of Epidemiology, 140*(5), 383–397.

Thacker, S. B., Choi, K., and Brachman, P. S. (1983). The surveillance of infectious diseases. *Journal of the American Medical Association, 249*(9), 1181–1185.

Tompkins, M. E. (1988). *Some preliminary thoughts on needs assessment.* Presentation at Region III Perinatal Information Consortium, Baltimore, MD.

Tribe, L. H. (1985). The abortion funding conundrum: Inalienable rights, affirmative duties, and the dilemma of dependence. *Harvard Law Review, 99*, 330–343.

Tudiver, F., Bass, M. J., Dunn, E. V., Norton, P. G., & Stewart, M. (Eds.). (1992). *Assessing interventions: Traditional and innovative methods.* Newbury Park, CA: Sage Publications.

Tugwell, P., Bennett, K. J., Sackett, D. L., and Haynes, R. B. (1985). The measurement iterative loop: A framework for the critical appraisal of need, benefits and cost of health interventions. *Journal of Chronic Diseases, 38*, 339–351.

United States Department of Health and Human Services.(1982). *Report to the Congress on the study of equitable formulas for the allocation of block grant runds for preventive health and health services, alcohol and drug abuse and mental health services, maternal and child health services.*

United States Department of Health and Human Services (1989). *Reducing the health consequences of smoking—25 years of progress: A report of the surgeon general.*

United Way of America. (1982). *Needs assessment. The state of the art: A guide for planners, managers, and funders of health and human care services.* Alexandria, VA: United Way of America, Planning and Allocations Division, United Way Institute.

Veblen-Mortenson, S. (1990). *A health-related needs assessment of the Washburn High School wellness center.* Plan B Submission for MPH in Community Health Education. Minneapolis: University of Minnesota School of Public Health (unpublished).

Wallace, H. M., Ryan, G., and Oglesby, A. C. (1988). *Maternal and child health practices* (3rd ed.). Oakland, CA: Third Party Publishing.

Wallace, H. M., Nelson, R. P., and Sweeney, P. J. (1994). *Maternal and child health practices* (4th ed.). Oakland CA: Third Party Publishing.

Warheit, G. J., Bell, R. A., and Schwab, J. J. (1977). *Needs assessment approaches: Concepts and methods.* Rockville, MD: Alcohol, Drug Abuse and Mental Health Administration.

Watcke, R. R. (1982). Community needs assessment: Using social indicators and key informants. *Community Services Catalyst, 12*(3), 6–10.

Welch, N. M. (1988). Benefits of community needs assessment. *American Journal of Public Health, 78*, 850–851.

Wilcox, L., and Marks, J. (Eds.). (1994). *From data to action: CDC's public health surveillance for women, infants and children.* Atlanta: Centers for Disease Control and Prevention, USDHHS.

Wilkin, D., Hallam, L., and Doggett, M. A. (1992). *Measures of need and outcome for primary health care.* New York: Oxford University Press.

Williams, D. R. (1997). Commentary on monitoring socioeconomic status. *Public Health Reports, 112*, 492–494.

Wilzack, A. (1988). *Department of health and mental hygiene report on funding formulas for the Family Health Administration.* Baltimore.

Wutchiett, R. (1991). *The "small area community health assessments projects."* Final Report: University of Connecticut School of Medicine and Connecticut State Department of Health Services.

Wutchiett, R., Egan, D., Kohaut, S., Markman, H. J., and Pargament, K. I. (1984). Assessing the need for a needs assessment. *Journal of Community Psychology, 12*: 53–59.

Index